Tips and Tricks in
Laparoscopic Urology

Udaya Kumar and
Inderbir S. Gill (*Editors*)

Tips and Tricks in Laparoscopic Urology

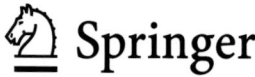 Springer

Udaya Kumar, MD, FRCS (Urol)
Associate Professor of
   Urology and Head
Section of Minimally
   Invasive Urology
University of Arkansas for
   Medical Sciences
Little Rock, AR, USA

Inderbir S. Gill, MD, MCh
Professor and Head
Section of Laparoscopic
   and Minimally Invasive
   Surgery
The Cleveland Clinic
Cleveland, OH, USA

British Library Cataloguing in Publication Data
A catalogue record for this book is available from the British Library

Library of Congress Control Number: 2006923492

ISBN-10: 1-84628-159-8   e-ISBN-10: 1-84628-160-1
ISBN-13: 978-1-84628-159-4   e-ISBN-13: 978-1-84628-160-0

Printed on acid-free paper

9 8 7 6 5 4 3 2 1

Springer Science+Business Media, LLC

Preface

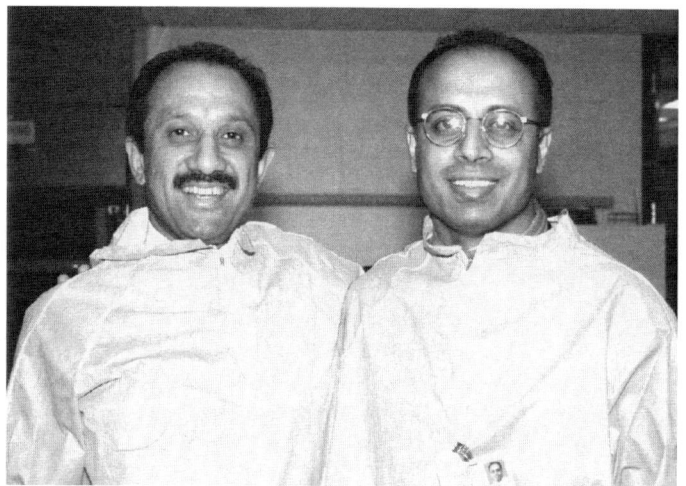

Surgical skills are learned by observation and apprenticeship over time. While most surgical textbooks describe the "standard" methods of performing a particular operation, all students of surgery are well aware that wide differences exist between surgeons in performing the same procedure or maneuver. The hallmark of a master surgeon is his/her ability to execute complex maneuvers with such aplomb as to make it appear the simplest and most effortless of tasks. Such skills are rarely described in books but infrequently appear as "points of technique" in journals. These "tips and tricks" are usually passed on from surgeon to surgeon, and only the fortunate few who have trained with or observed an expert surgeon get to learn the critical techniques that can make a difficult procedure easier, safer, and more efficient. These tips and tricks of master surgeons therefore have benefitted only those they have trained. This compilation of tips and tricks represents our desire to make such knowledge available to the laparoscopic urological community at large.

Laparoscopic urology has witnessed the introduction of various procedures that were practically nonexistent only a few years ago. There is a desire among more and more residents and practicing urologists to acquire laparoscopic skills and become proficient. This book brings together the viewpoints of talented urologic laparoscopic surgeons from around the world. We asked them how they performed not only complex urologic procedures but also basic steps of surgery such as patient positioning or insertion of the Veress needle. We have intentionally sought out several surgeons' contrasting viewpoints on the same procedure or maneuver to demonstrate to the reader the array of options available for handling a given situation. After all, there are many ways to "skin a prostate"!

The editors are grateful to the contributors—all of whom are internationally respected for their laparoscopic expertise—for their time, effort, and willingness to share their experience. We hope that the reader will learn as much from reading this handbook as we did in talking with these expert surgeons.

Udaya Kumar MS, FRCS (Urol)
Associate Professor of Urology
Director of Minimally Invasive Urology
University of Arkansas for Medical Sciences
Little Rock, Arkansas
USA

Inderbir S. Gill MD, MCh
Professor and Head, Section of Laparoscopic and
Minimally Invasive Surgery
Cleveland, Ohio
USA

Contents

Contributing Authors

David M. Albala, MD
Professor of Urology
Duke University Medical Center
Durham, North Carolina, USA

Gary C. Bellman, MD
Residency Program Director, Urology
Kaiser Foundation Hospital
Los Angeles, California, USA

Jeffery A. Cadeddu, MD
Associate Professor
Department of Urology
UT Southwestern Medical Center
Dallas, Texas, USA

Jean de la Rosette, MD, PhD
Professor and Chairman
Department of Urology
Academic Medical Center
Amsterdam, The Netherlands

Mihir M. Desai, MD
Glickman Urological Institute
The Cleveland Clinic Foundation
Cleveland, Ohio, USA

Christopher G. Eden, MBBS, MS, FRCS (Urol)
Consultant Urological Surgeon
The North Hampshire Hospital
Basingstoke, UK

Matthew Gettman, MD
Urology Consultant
Mayo Clinic
Rochester, Minnesota, USA

Alaa El-Ghoneimi, MD, PhD
Professor of Pediatric Surgery, University of Paris VII
Hôpital Robert Debré
Paris, France

Inderbir S. Gill, MD, MCh
Head, Section of Laparoscopic and Robotic Surgery
Glickman Urological Institute
The Cleveland Clinic Foundation
Cleveland, Ohio, USA

Jihad H. Kaouk, MD
Co-Director, Robotic Urologic Surgery
Glickman Urological Institute
The Cleveland Clinic Foundation
Cleveland, Ohio, USA

Francis X. Keeley, MD, FRCS Urol
Consultant Urologist
Bristol Urological Institute
Westbury-on-Trym, UK

Udaya Kumar, MD, FRCS Urol
Associate Professor and Head, Section of Minimally
Invasive Urology
University of Arkansas for Medical Sciences
Little Rock, Arkansas, USA

M. Pilar Laguna, MD, PhD
Department of Urology
Academic Medical Center, University of Amsterdam
The Netherlands

Albert A. Mikhail, MD
Minimally Invasive Surgery Fellow
Department of Surgery, Section of Urology
University of Chicago
Chicago, Illinois, USA

Stephen Y. Nakada, MD
Professor and Chairman of Urology
University of Wisconsin
Madison, Wisconsin, USA

Yoshinari Ono, MD, PhD
Professor of Urology
Nagoya University Graduate School of Medicine
Nagoya-shi, Japan

Jens Rassweiler, MD
Professor of Urology
SLK Kliniken Heilbronn
Heilbronn, Germany

Arieh L. Shalhav, MD
Vice Chief, Section of Urology, Head of Minimally
Invasive Surgery
Department of Surgery, Section of Urology
University of Chicago
Chicago, Illinois, USA

Andrew I. Shpall, MD
Endourology Fellow
Kaiser Foundation Hospital
Los Angeles, California, USA

Marshall L. Stoller, MD
Professor and Vice Chairman
Department of Urology
University of California San Francisco
San Francisco, California, USA

Li-Ming Su, MD
Assistant Professor of Urology
Director of Pelvic Laparoscopy
Brady Urological Institute, Johns Hopkins
Baltimore, Maryland, USA

Kazuo Suzuki, MD
Professor of Urology
Hamamatsu University School of Medicine
Hamamatsu, Japan

Raju Thomas, MD, FACS, MHA
Professor and Chairman
Department of Urology
Tulane University Health Sciences Center
New Orleans, Louisiana, USA

J. Stuart Wolf, MD
Director, Division of Minimally Invasive Urology
University of Michigan Medical Center
Ann Arbor, Michigan, USA

Chapter 1
General Laparoscopic Tips

How Do You Organize Your Foot Pedals for the Various Energy Sources?

Dr. Udaya Kumar

Monopolar diathermy, bipolar diathermy, Harmonic scalpel, and argon beam coagulator are some of the most commonly used energy sources during laparoscopic surgery, often all during the same case. This creates a clutter of foot pedals on the floor near the surgeon. One trick to reduce this clutter is to tape the smaller bipolar diathermy pedal securely onto the top of the monopolar diathermy pedal, which is taped to the floor. The current model of the Harmonic scalpel is entirely hand-activated, eliminating the need for a foot pedal.

How about Patient Positioning?

Dr. Kumar

For transperitoneal nephrectomy, I position the patient in a 45- to 60-degree lateral position. For retroperitoneal nephrectomy a full flank position is used. Align the iliac crest at the flexion point of the table to achieve adequate opening of the space between the iliac crest and the 12th rib for retroperitoneal procedures. We take care to minimize the degree of table flexion and only minimally elevate the kidney rest. This is important to prevent neuromuscular injuries and rhabdomyolysis, which can be severe issues.

During laparoscopic radical prostatectomy, the patient is positioned in a steep Trendelenberg position. The patient tends to slide toward the head end of the bed when maintained in this position for prolonged periods of time. There are several suggestions to overcome this difficulty. One we have found most useful is to place the patient (with no intervening gown, clothing or other material) on flat gel padding. This provides adequate traction to prevent the patient from sliding. An X-shaped tape, from below each shoulder across the chest, taped to the bed is also useful. Using shoulder guards to buttress each shoulder is a bad idea as the patient can develop pressure-induced neuropraxia.

Dr. David Albala

For the positioning during nephrectomy, I like to use a beanbag. I position the patient with an axillary roll in a modified flank position with arms folded. The beanbag allows one to position the patient adequately and after it is deflated, the patient is securely held in that position. I don't think that the kidney rest adds anything to patient positioning for this procedure.

How Do You Organize Your Laparoscopic Instruments?

Dr. Kumar

The array of instruments that one uses during laparoscopy also causes a clutter on the instrument

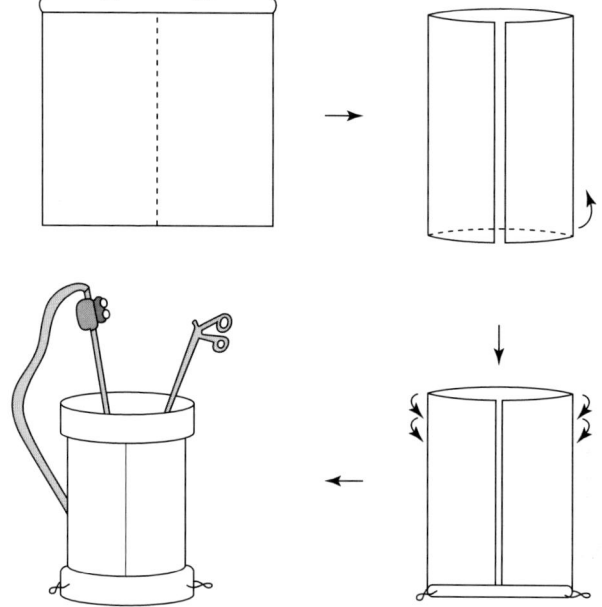

Fig. 1.1 Instrument holder.

table. One way to circumvent this is by using two or three instrument holders that will conveniently hold four to five instruments each. The holders are strategically placed within easy reach of the surgeon.

The instrument holder is made simply by using a small sterile towel that is commonly available. The towel is folded twice toward the middle. One end of the towel is closed off by folding and clipping with a towel clip. The open end is turned inside out twice, creating a collar. The instrument holder is ready! One may not only hold any of the long laparoscopic instruments with this pouch but also the hot water flask that is used for warming up the laparoscope lens.

Your Thoughts about Starting with Laparoscopy?

Dr. Jean de la Rosette

One of the problems faced by people starting to get involved in laparoscopy is that they have difficulty making choices. They move from one technique where they see an improvement to the next and then the next and the next. What I would strongly recommend when starting out with laparoscopy is that, first of all, mentoring is very important. The way we learned all the tricks is that one of my colleagues went away for half a year for training elsewhere, where he participated actively in laparoscopic surgery. That same colleague committed himself, for one year, to come to our place, once every week (for training) and then we continued learning the tips and tricks from him for the next one or two years till we became good at them. Only then did we shift to a higher level and change small things here and there. It is always good to have a strict schedule and not to try to improve too fast while one is not yet familiar with the technology.

What Is Your Typical Bowel Preparation for Laparoscopic Surgery?

Dr. Inderbir Gill

I believe in the dictum that "an empty colon is a happy colon." As such, typically, for all laparoscopic surgery, unless there is a contraindication, I request the patient to take two bottles of magnesium citrate on the afternoon prior to surgery, with nil orally from midnight. This is pretty much true for all abdominal laparoscopic surgery in an adult. For laparoscopic radical cystectomy wherein bowel urinary diversion is anticipated, a more thorough bowel preparation comprising 4 liters of Go-Lytely® and a Fleets® enema the evening before surgery is performed. We typically do not perform antibiotic preparation of the bowel. Clearly, different surgeons have different protocols for bowel preparation during laparoscopic surgery.

How Do You Position the Patient's Arms during Various Urologic Laparoscopic Procedures?

Dr. Gill

For all pelvic laparoscopic surgeries (prostatectomy, radical cystectomy, pelvic lymph node dissection, incontinence surgery, seminal vesical surgery, etc.), both arms are carefully padded and adducted by the patient's side. This is important since outstretched arms severely limit the surgeon's own mobility, and may also lead to hyperextension of the arms and brachial plexus injury. For renal and adrenal laparoscopy, wherein the patient is placed in the flank position, the standard arm positioning, similar to open surgery in the flank position, is obtained. Care must be taken to appropriately pad the axilla, and all bony prominences, maintaining extremities in a neutral position.

Do You Apply Local Anesthetic at Port Sites?

Dr. Stuart Wolf

We are impressed by the effectiveness of bupivacaine infiltration at port sites for reducing pain after laparoscopy. We published a randomized trial in the *Journal of Urology* that demonstrated bupivacaine infiltration to reduce narcotic use by almost 50%, and the results were statistically significant in both standard transperitoneal laparoscopic and hand-assisted laparoscopic sub-groups.[1] At the beginning of the case, we infiltrate 0.5% bupivacaine into the pre-peritoneal tissues at the port sites, and for hand-assisted cases we also infiltrate the fascia around the incision for the hand-assistance device. The total amount is 30 ml, divided up between the various sites (5–10 ml in port sites, and 15 ml at the hand-assistance site).

Any Tips for Obtaining Abdominal Entry for Laparoscopic Surgery?

Dr. Matthew Gettman

The one thing about entering the abdomen that I like to do, especially during placement of the first trocar is, after

I have made my 1-cm incision, I use trachea hooks and I anchor the trachea hooks into the fascia as opposed to using towel clamps. It really anchors the abdominal wall during placement of the initial trocar and I usually use a closed (Veress needle) technique. This technique of using the trachea hook was something that I learned from Reinhardt Peschel and Gunter Janetschek in Austria.

Dr. Pilar Laguna

We place our first port (for the laparoscope) in an open fashion and after opening the fascia, we immediately place a fascial stitch. During exit, we have the fascial stitch already in place and closure is more rapid (Figure 1.2).

Also to avoid leakage of gas if the incision of the first port is slightly bigger than 12 mm, we place a small piece of Tul Grasum (or a small gauze with Vaseline) under the skin and around the trocar (Figure 1.3).

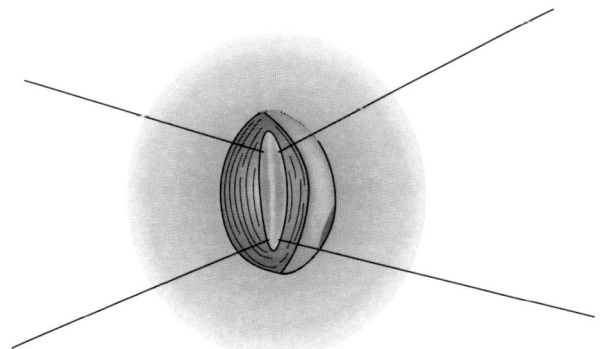

Fig. 1.2 Fascial stitch at entry.

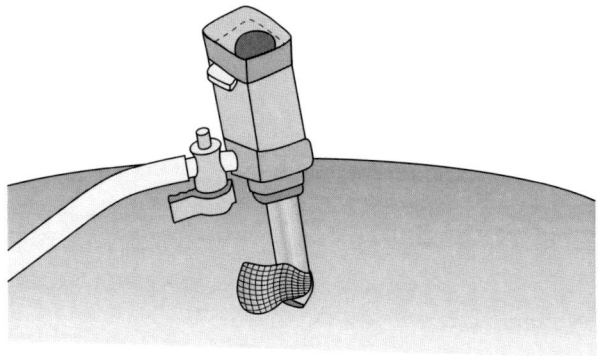

Fig. 1.3 Vaseline gauze to prevent air leak.

What Is Your Technique for Veress Needle Insertion and Trocar Placement?

Dr. Marshall Stoller

A trick that I use is our initial blind Veress access. We have now done over 700 laparoscopic upper tract procedures and we always use Palmer's point, which is one fingerbreadth below the costal margin at the lateral border of the rectus muscle (Figure 1.4). Palmer described it on the left side; we do a congruent puncture site on the right side. Even with previous abdominal operations, needle placement is very unlikely to encounter adhesions or cause bowel injuries in these locations. When we do a pelvic procedure, we will still go up high at Palmer's point for initial access and establish pneumoperitoneum. We've never had a splenic injury on the left side. On occasion we have had a punc-

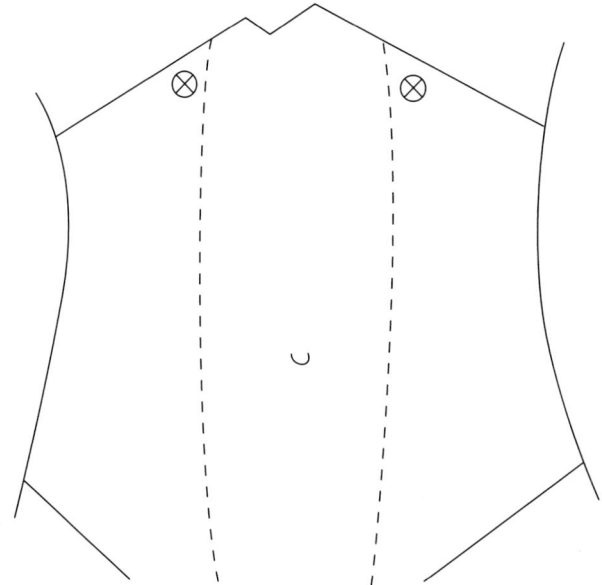

Fig. 1.4 Palmer's point.

ture hole in the liver on the right, but there has been no need for any intervention in those cases, although one should always keep this foremost in mind.

Dr. Kazuo Suzuki

In general, I prefer to insert the first trocar by the open technique. If using the Veress needle technique, I like to use the 2-mm telescope inserted through the Veress needle port to place other trocars under direct laparoscopic observation, avoiding bowel or other visceral injury.

Dr. de la Rosette

One tip only: don't use the Veress needle! Just go for an open access. In my opinion, it is safer. It is easier and faster.

Dr. Gill

Almost always, I use the Veress needle. . . . In over 4,000 cases, we have used the Veress needle predominantly, even in patients with history of previous abdominal surgery. Everybody does it differently; and this is how I do it. There are a number of little, little steps that one should go through every time one uses the Veress needle. First, make sure that the needle is patent, by injecting saline through it. Second, make sure that its spring-loaded blunt tip is working well. Select an appropriate site in the abdomen, distant from any previous surgical incisions and make a skin stab incision which will easily admit the needle tip without the skin catching on the needle. Make sure that the insufflation is low (one liter per minute), with maximum insufflation pressure (20 mm Hg). Holding the needle in mid-shaft like a dart or a pen, insert the needle vertically at right angle to the skin. Some surgeons prefer to grab or pinch the anterior abdominal wall and lift it up in an attempt to increase the distance between the abdominal wall and the abdominal viscera. However, we believe this is counterproductive. The only thing that this maneuver achieves is lifting up the subcutaneous fat, thereby actually increasing the distance between the skin and the peritoneum, which itself stays in relatively the same position. As such, we believe that this maneuver actually increases the degree of difficulty of Veress needle insertion. The Veress needle should be inserted gently with the abdominal wall in neutral position, being on the look out for two distinct pops, one for the fascia and the second for the peritoneum. The drop test is then done (aspirate, inject 5 cc and re-aspirate) to evaluate the needle-tip position. Finally, easy egress of the drop in the needle into the abdominal cavity under gravity is a good sign. However, none of these tests are fail proof. The one thing never to do is to move the needle in a circular manner to evaluate freedom of its tip in the abdomen. Obviously, this can cause critical and grievous injury to internal abdominal organs and blood vessels. Thereafter, insufflation is started at a low flow state as mentioned above. Initial pressures should be less than 10 to 12 mm Hg. Also, generalized tympany should result rather than asymmetric localized tympany, which indicates that the needle tip is in the wrong place. Once low pressures and generalized tympany have been confirmed, the flow rate is then increased to maximum.

How Does One Get Laparoscopic Access into a Previously Operated Abdomen?

Dr. Gill

There are essentially three ways to go about it. First, if transperitoneal laparoscopy is intended, you can go in with the open (Hassan) technique, where an open cut-down is made for placement of the primary port. In this manner, the planned port is placed under vision, thereby minimizing access-related injury. However, it's important to keep in mind that even with the open technique you can still create a bowel injury; it has been reported in the literature. The second option for transperitoneal access would be to perform close entry with a Veress needle, my preferred approach. However, significant prior laparoscopic expertise is necessary before one undertakes this. The important point in this regard is to select the quadrant in the abdomen which is furthest away from the abdominal scar. So, for example, if a patient has had an appendectomy with the scar in the right iliac fossa, the initial Veress needle entry should be in the right or left hypochondrium. I would prefer the right, because on the left side, one can potentially cause a Veress injury of the spleen, which is a serious injury. The third option is to avoid the peritoneal cavity completely, and perform the procedure by the retroperitoneal laparoscopic technique. However, adequate expertise with retroperitoneal laparoscopy is essential. Another option would be to obtain retroperitoneal access, put in the laparoscope, and then under vision, create a large peritoneotomy and put in the transperitoneal ports under retroperitoneoscopic visualization, and finally convert to a completely transperitoneal procedure.

Dr. Raju Thomas

We now perform advanced laparoscopic procedures, sometimes in patients with previous abdominal surgery, such as ileostomy, colostomy, or following other surgical procedures. Tricks used to stay out of trouble, if you get an off-site access, are—

1. If the previous incision is in the mid-line, for example, you enter on the side and location of the abdomen furthest away from the previous incision;

2. I only use a blunt trocar system to gain access. I prefer the Step® trocars. Once you know you are in the right place, after placing your laparoscope, if there are no adhesions, you are lucky. However, in most cases you are faced with adhesions. What we recommend at this stage is to use the teaching laparoscope, which is an off-set laparoscope and has a working channel similar to an off-set nephroscope (Figure 1.5). I use the working channel of the off-set laparoscope to dissect myself out of these adhesions and get enough working space through a single port without having to place additional ports. I use the laparoscopic scissors through the working channel of the teaching off-set laparoscope to gain space and then I am able to place

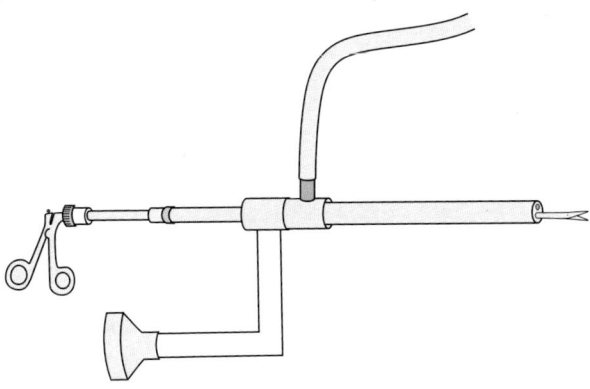

Fig. 1.5 Operating laparoscope.

a second working port. This is a trick I have found very useful.

How Do You Achieve Port Placement for Transperitoneal Surgery?

Dr. Wolf

Port placements are always very hard to convey from one surgeon to the next, even with diagrams. Describing them relative to anatomical landmarks is more helpful than using absolute terms. For a hand-assisted nephrectomy, I put my primary 12-mm port one or two fingerbreadths lateral to the hand-assistance device, given my typical peri-umbilical incision for the hand-assistance device. The 12-mm working port is placed on a line from the primary port toward the ipsilateral shoulder, approximately two fingerbreadths below the costal margin. This reference gets the working port in the right spot on most occasions, regardless of patient morphology (with the exception of very obese patients, where the hand-assistance device is placed more cephalad and lateral). I like to have a third port, 5 mm, for all cases—it allows the assistant to provide counter traction. The placement of this port is less critical, as long as it is caudal to the primary port and lateral to the working port (Figure 1.6). For a standard transperitoneal laparoscopic nephrectomy, the primary port is placed on the lateral edge of the rectus abdominis muscle in line with the umbilicus. For the working and assisting ports I again advocate relative rather than absolute port placements. Here, draw

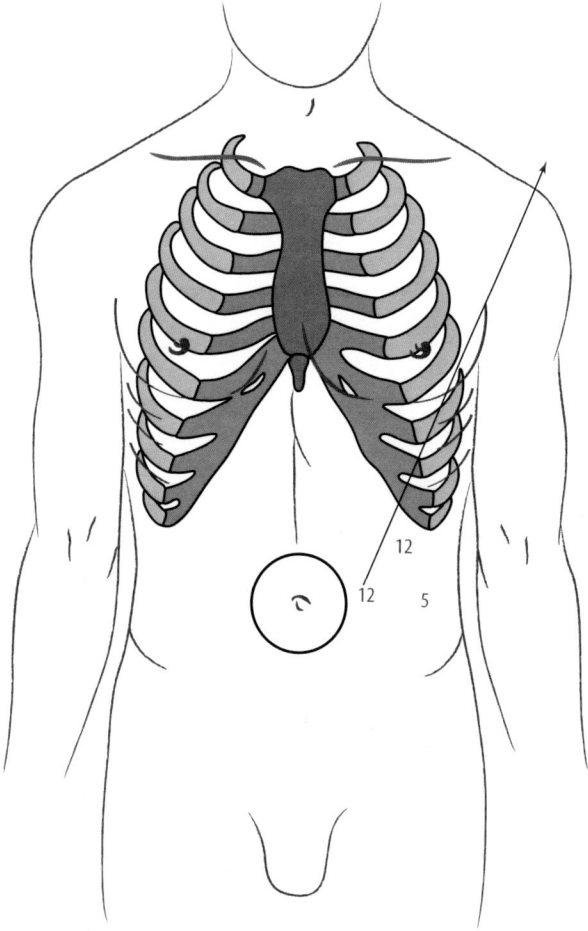

Fig. 1.6 Port placement for hand-assisted nephrectomy.

a line from the xiphoid process to the anterior superior iliac spine. Three ports are placed along this line: cephalad, on the border of the rectus sheath (5 mm); caudal, slightly below the level of the primary port (5 mm); and one in between these 2 ports (12 mm) (Figure 1.7).

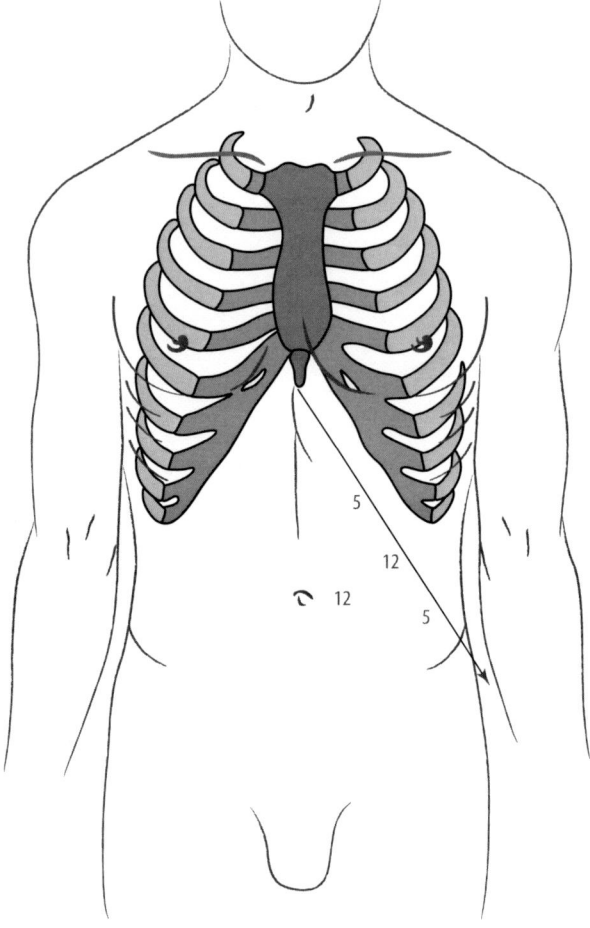

Fig. 1.7 Port placement for transperitoneal nephrectomy.

When Using the Retroperitoneal Approach, What Do You Do in Cases When the Space Between the Iliac Crest and the Lower Ribs is Very Narrow?

Dr. Jens Rassweiler

There are two points. The space usually opens up when you inflate the retroperitoneal space with Carbon Dioxide. The second point is that a supra-costal port might make sense. If we are going to use the supra-costal port primarily, then we would put the lower port first, trying to create space and then placing the supra-costal port under vision. I don't use the balloon; to me it is not necessary. I dissect just with a finger and complete the rest of the dissection with instruments.

How Does One Optimize Port Placement during Retroperitoneoscopy?

Dr. Gill

"Crowding" of ports can be a significant problem during retroperitoneal laparoscopy. As such, adequate spacing of ports is essential. The primary port holding the laparoscope is typically placed at the tip of the twelfth rib. I always create the retroperitoneal space with balloon dilation—it is rapid, easy, and standardized: even the fellows and residents can learn easily. Balloon dilation has taken the mystique out of retroperitoneal laparoscopy, which is a good thing. Once balloon dilation has been completed, ports are placed. Two secondary ports are placed, one at the angle of the erector spinae muscle and the 12th rib, and the second at the anterior axillary line approximately two to three fingerbreadths cephalad to the anterior superior iliac spine (Figure 1.8). Typically, this results in the three ports' being placed in a straight oblique line along the undersurface of the twelfth rib with enough separation that virtually no crowding of ports occurs. Again, typically for all retroperitoneal renal and adrenal surgery, these three ports' are employed. Occasionally, an additional 5-mm port is placed anteriorly at the tip of the 11th rib (for partial nephrectomy) to provide traction on the renal parenchymal sutures. All retroperitoneal ports are placed under clear laparoscopic visualization. In our experience, this port placement is efficacious, and we have not experienced the problem of "clashing of swords."

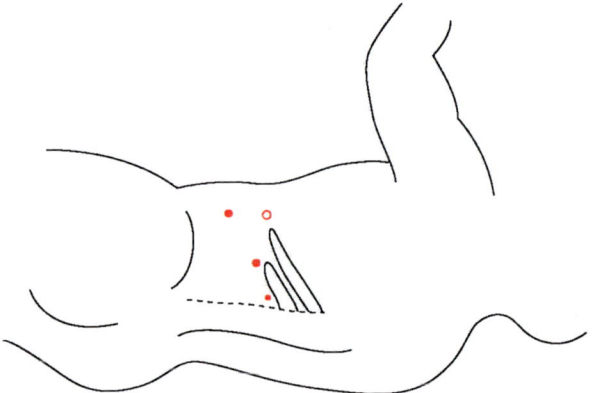

Fig. 1.8 Port placement for retroperitoneal laparoscopy.

Dr. Kumar

One of the problems I face during port placement for retroperitoneal laparoscopic surgery is that the space between the iliac crest and 12th rib never seems adequate! Unlike transperitoneal surgery, where ports can be placed as far away from one another as one likes, one often finds that the space between the lower ribs and the iliac crest is limited, despite flexion of the operating table. Placement of the first port just below the tip of the 12th rib is often the standard approach, followed by a port at the angle between the 12th rib and the paraspinal musculature. Another port is usually placed a few fingerbreadths above the iliac crest in the anterior axillary line.

I have changed these port placements following the advice of Dr. Klaus Jeschke from Austria based on his impressive series of laparoscopic partial nephrectomy cases, all done through the retroperitoneal route. I now place the first port in the angle between the 12th rib and the paraspinal muscles. After balloon dilatation and confirming good placement, I remove the balloon and place the next two ports by palpation, one a few fingerbreadths above the iliac crest and the other supero-medial to the tip of the 12th rib or even above the 11th rib if the space appears very crowded. Despite the theoretical risk of creating pneumothorax when a port is placed above the 11th rib, the risk is minimal when the port is placed anterior to the anterior axillary line.

I use the port between the 12th rib and spinal muscles for the camera (rather than the tip of the 12th rib port as I used to earlier) as I believe this provides a more direct view of the renal hilum and ease of dissection.

Can One Introduce a Needle through a 5-mm Port?

Dr. Francis Keeley

A very simple and seemingly minor tip would be introducing an SH needle through a 5-mm port, which I learned from David E. McGinnis from Thomas Jefferson University Hospital in Philadelphia. Take the free tail end of the suture away from the needle and introduce that through a port. Grasp it with another grasper or needle holder inside the abdomen; pull the needle holder out through the port so that the needle is going in through the port alone. Then drag the needle through the port from the inside. That way you can use nothing but 5-mm ports for a laparoscopic pyeloplasty. Some people find that they need a larger port so they can get a needle in and out and I don't think that is necessary.

Righting the Needle on a Needle Holder Using One Hand

Dr. Keeley

Trying to position a needle on a needle driver can be a frustrating part of the suturing technique. One should find a fairly firm surface such as the kidney or psoas muscle and then loosen the grip slightly on the needle while holding it in the center of the needle. Pushing down into the kidney or psoas will tend to make the needle face up as a smile and so it tends to right the needle into the needle holder. Of course it takes a little bit of practice but this is preferable to handing the needle back and forth between two needle holders which can bend the needle or just cause frustration. Oftentimes, this is something that you can do with one needle holder, which again is an advantage if you have some tissue in the grasper in the other hand which you would rather not let go.

What Is Your Technique of Specimen Entrapment?

Dr. Wolf

Entrapping the kidney using the LapSac® (Cook Urologic, Spender, IN) for morcellation can be a miserable experience, even with the trick of placing a wire into the holes of the bag to make it somewhat self-opening. With the original morcellation technique described by Clayman, the durable LapSac,® rather than a self-opening but flimsy retrieval bag such as the Endocatch,® must be used in cases of morcellation, because the flimsy bag can be ripped by the morcellator (clamp) very easily. When the self-opening bag was used, which greatly simplifies entrapment, it was thought that the specimen removal had to be intact. Jamie Landman described a great technique that provides the best of both worlds— safe morcellation but in the easy-to-use self-opening bag.[2] After entrapping the specimen in the self-opening bag, bring the neck of the bag back up through the port site, and then enlarge the incision just enough so that you can actually see within the bag. Then you grab and morcellate only the tissue that you can see; it is a more rapid process because you can remove bigger pieces. You are not blindly morcellating, which would be unsafe in a flimsy plastic bag, but rather you are morcellating under vision. Dr. Landman's data suggested that this was safe, and our experience is similar. For most patients you are only going to enlarge that incision to about 2.5 to 3 cm wide. If you had started with a 12-mm diameter port at that site, the length of the skin incision is 18 mm (assuming that the skin did not stretch). So you have added about 50% to the length of the small incision, and now you can easily entrap the specimen and then morcellate quickly under direct vision. I doubt if most patients are bothered by the extra 7 to 12 mm on one incision.

How Do You Exit the Abdomen?

Dr. Laguna

We have found the Bercy needle (or similar) extremely useful to place the fascial stitches under vision before desufflating the abdominal cavity.

Do You Perform Fascial Closure of the Port Sites after Retroperitoneoscopy?

Dr. Wolf

I rarely do intact extraction in association with retroperitoneoscopy, and as a result am faced with the challenge of closing the fascia through a 2-cm primary port site incision. Following a retroperitoneoscopic radical nephrectomy on a morbidly obese patient, the fascia may be more than 5 cm deep, and working through a shorter (2 cm) incision to close from the outside is very challenging. A needle-suture passer such as the Carter-Thomason device is unwieldy to use under laparoscopic guidance in the small working space of retroperitoneoscopy, especially since the incision is too large to close with a simple suture and either a pair of sutures or a figure-of-eight suture is needed. We've learned to do it with finger-guidance (Figure 1.9). Looking back at the primary port site from the most medial port (a 5-mm 30-degree lens will be needed, if there are only 5-mm ports medially), the closure device can be directed with a finger down through the fat and to catch a generous bite of the lumbodorsal fascia. The suture is dropped off, the device is removed and reinserted on the other side, and the suture is grasped and pulled out to complete the first half of a figure-of-eight suture. This technique has allowed us to close these fascial defects through 2-cm skin incisions, which otherwise would have been very hard to close without opening the skin incision for visualization. Before we figured this out, we gave up closing the fascia on a few obese patients, and at least 2 patients (of approximately 30 until we altered our technique) developed flank hernias at the site.

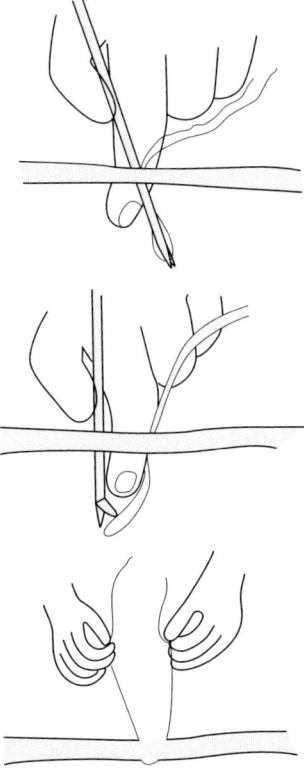

Fig. 1.9 Finger-guided use of the Carter–Thomason device.

What Are Your Favorite Instruments?

Dr. Suzuki

The combined suction/irrigation/ electro-cautery device can be used for dissection also. Often, it is useful to perform suction and dissection simultaneously with this device. Nowadays, we have started using the electro-cautery hook on 80–100 W power. This is very high power indeed, but if one is careful, it provides a nice tool for dissection. In areas such as the posterior surface of the kidney, where there are few important structures, one can use it effectively. I have observed Dr. Menon use such high-power (120 W) cautery in robotic laparoscopic radical prostatectomy very effectively, and I have adopted this technique in my surgery also. (Editors' note: The editors do not recommend monopolar coagulation at settings above 55 W as they believe that higher settings increase the potential for unrecognized thermal injury to bowel).

Dr. Gill

For renal and adrenal surgery, I typically like to use the atraumatic small bowel grasper in my left hand for retraction and exposure purposes and variably use the right angle J-hook monopolar electrode, the Stryker smooth suction tip, or laparoscopic endoshears in my right hand (I am right-handed). During prostatectomy, the left hand typically holds the small bowel grasper or the locking Allis clamp while the right hand typically employs the J-hook or the Harmonic scalpel. For suturing, I prefer the Ethicon® straight-locking 5-mm needle driver.

Dr. Yoshinari Ono

My favorite instrument is the "D" retractor, the one that forms like a circle within the abdomen. The coat-hanger type retractor is a little too large. The "D" retractor is more round. Also, functionally it is very important for removal of the lymph nodes. For dissection we usually use the ultrasonic scissors and the curved dissecting forceps.

Dr. Stoller

Everyone asks what instruments you would take with you if you had to perform a procedure outside your own hospital. We all have our favorite instruments. The cigarette sponge is one of mine. The laparoscopic cigarette-sponge (Kittner Rolled Gauze—Carefree Surgical Specialties, Inc., 450 Main St. New Castle, CA 95658, ph. 916-663-4082) is a key tool for multiple aspects of laparoscopy. It is a pre-rolled 4 × 4 gauze with umbilical tape that does not get stuck on the valves of the laparoscopy port. They come in sets of five and are very useful.

First, you can place this sponge through a 10-mm port. It is easier to soak up peritoneal fluid, lymph, urine, or blood with a sponge than to utilize suction that decreases the pneumoperitoneal pressure and decreases the image quality. If there is bothersome oozing, you can pack it with a sponge and leave it there, just as you would in open surgery, and then come back later to address it. You can use it on a grasper just as a sponge on a stick is used in open surgery, to help with blunt dissection of the colon. During a difficult nephrectomy where you are trying to define the anterior and the posterior aspect of the dissection, placing a cigarette-sponge behind or in front of the hilum as you flip the kidney back and forth (as with a donor nephrectomy) allows you to have an idea of how much further your dissection needs to go. You can also estimate how much blood loss you have. You can take them out and squeeze them to get an idea of how much blood is there.

An important aspect is to be sure that you remove all the sponges you put in. We will frequently have put ten sponges in at a time to help with packing. You must keep track of where those sponges are. If you are doing a donor nephrectomy or morcellating a kidney, it is important to take the sponges out before you start to remove the specimens. They will be difficult to find after the loss of the pneumoperitoneum. Cigarette sponges have a radio-opaque marker woven in them, so if there is a question of inability to find one, you can get an x-ray. I think the cigarette sponge is something everyone should use.

Dr. Kumar

I find the long packing gauze (Fabco ORS, First Aid Bandage Co. Old Mystic, CT) particularly useful to absorb blood or other fluid, as well act as a tamponade if bothersome ooze occurs during dissection. Since it is available in 0.5- and 1-inch widths, the gauze can be cut to the required length and easily inserted through one of the ports. As it comes with a radio-opaque marker, it is easy to locate radiographically should it become necessary. With hand-assisted laparoscopy, of course, it is easy to place a large lap sponge through the hand incision.

What Are Some Tips on Minimizing Costs for Laparoscopic Surgery?

Dr. Jeffrey Cadeddu

The most important things are, of course, comfort in doing the procedure and the patient's safety and a good outcome. As one develops experience, I believe there are ways to reduce the cost of the procedures in every aspect of the operation. Beginning with access and trocars, one can obviously use reusable trocars and that reduces cost. In terms of doing the dissection, I do not use the harmonic scalpel for any of my procedures, though it is advocated by some, particularly general surgeons, because it adds a $300 cost to every operation. For such cases as nephrectomy, I don't see how a harmonic scalpel is very useful. One just has to be more meticulous in application of bipolar or monopolar energy in the dissection rather than just cutting through, slowly, with the harmonic scalpel. Other means of reducing cost is in the technology used for hemostasis. I have switched now to Hem-O-Lok® clips whenever possible. Not necessarily because they are more efficacious than regular clips but because they cost about 60% less than metal clips and so it is also a significant way of reducing cost. Postoperatively it is pretty clear that it is beneficial to avoid narcotics, which can contribute to a slightly longer time to return of bowel function and so necessitate a longer postoperative hospital stay. Preparing the patient psychologically for going home the next day and early return of bowel function by using nonsteroidal anti-inflammatories for pain are the most important perioperative factors.

How Does One Retract the Liver and the Spleen during Renal or Adrenal Laparoscopic Surgery?

Dr. Gill

In my view, the safest and best way to retract the liver is to retract from medial to the lateral side. In other words, the instrument retracting the liver should be inserted high in the midline of the abdomen near the xiphisternum and carefully passed along the undersurface of the liver towards the lateral sidewall. Care must be taken to avoid injury to the gall bladder. Various instruments can be used to retract the liver, e.g., fan-retractor, "snake-retractor," etc. However, we have found that the simplest way to achieve this is by using a locking Allis 5-mm clamp inserted through a high midline port near the xiphisternum, passed under the liver, to grasp the lateral abdominal wall at a desired location. The Allis clamp is then closed and locked, thereby creating a self-retaining retractor that does not require an assistant to hold it (Figure 1.10). It stays out of the way and keeps the liver adequately retracted. On rare occasions when the liver is extremely large, two such graspers can be passed through ports placed adjacent to each other. Caution: retracting the liver using an instrument passed from lateral to medial or from an instrument passed from an inferiorly placed port is dangerous. The angle of retraction of the liver is inadequate from such a direction, and there is a real danger of lacerating the liver.

As regards the spleen, there is no good way to retract the spleen adequately during a left-sided renal/adrenal

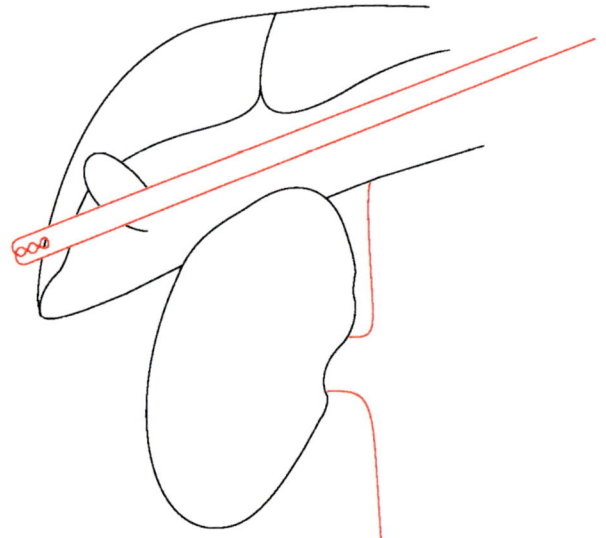

Fig. 1.10 Retraction of liver using an Allis locking clamp.

laparoscopic procedure. The best thing to do is to mobilize the spleen as thoroughly as is safe and feasible. While mobilizing the spleen, care must be taken not to tear the splenic capsule or to injure the diaphragm. Further, as the lateral peritoneal incision around the spleen is developed cephalad, one can occasionally run into the greater curvature of the stomach, which should be guarded against. In our experience, extensive and high mobilization of the spleen is readily performed laparoscopically, similar to open surgery. Care must be taken to do this slowly. Excellent hemostasis must be achieved every step of the way, since one is typically working at the very extreme of the instruments' length. Not infrequently, despite such extensive mobilization of the spleen, it still is in the way while performing dissection of the renal hilum. The safest way to retract the mobilized spleen medially is to insert a 10/12-mm port in the suprapubic area, low down on the abdomen. A 4 × 18 lap sponge is inserted, the pancreas and spleen carefully padded, and then a three-pronged standard fan retractor is inserted through this suprapubic port to retract the padded structures medially. Medial retraction of the spleen with an instrument inserted through a lateral port is extremely dangerous and has a high chance of causing splenic injury.

How Do You Select the Appropriate Suture for Laparoscopic Suturing?

Dr. Gill

Selection of the laparoscopic suture depends on the color, texture, memory, and length of the suture and the shape and size of the needle (Figure 1.11). A laparoscopic suture should be easily visible laparoscopically. It should have minimal coil memory. It should be easy to handle laparoscopically. It should not have excess length, which leads to unnecessary intertwining within the abdomen, significantly increasing the level of technical difficulty. From a personal standpoint, the dyed (violet) Vicryl® or Monocryl® are desirable sutures for laparoscopic surgery. Conversely, a Prolene® suture is much more difficult to handle. Typically, the suture is cut to the length of the port, which is usually long enough for most laparoscopic suturing, while still being readily manageable. With regard to needles, different shapes and sizes

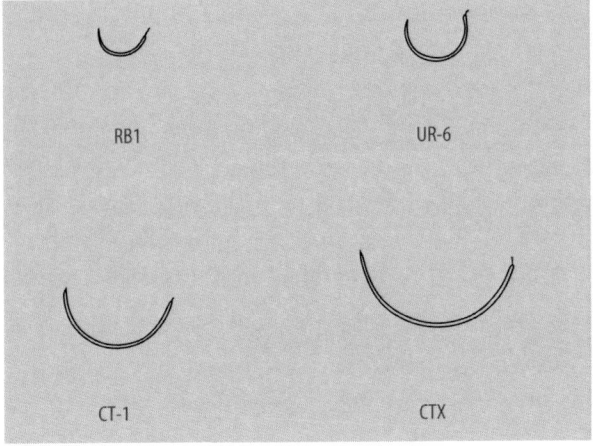

Fig. 1.11 Selection of needles for laparoscopic suturing.

of needles are required for different suturing situations. Furthermore, needle preferences vary according to the individual surgeon. Personally speaking, a UR-6 needle is optimal for the urethrovesical anastomosis during laparoscopic radical prostatectomy because of its 58th curve, allowing ease of handling. Typically, we employ a 2–0 Vicryl® suture on a UR-6 needle for the urethrovesical anastomosis. The same applies for the urethro-ileal anastomosis of a laparoscopic orthotopic neobladder. For dorsal vein ligation, we employ a CT-1 needle on 2–0 Vicryl. The same stitch is used for laparoscopic bowel suturing. For laparoscopic uretero-intestinal anastomosis, we employ an RB-1 needle on 4–0 Vicryl. This is the same stitch that is employed for laparoscopic dismembered pyeloplasty. During laparoscopic partial nephrectomy, we employ a CT-1 needle with 2–0 Vicryl for watertight suture-repair of the pelvic calicyeal system and parenchymal suturing for hemostasis. For renal parenchymal re-approximation over a bolster, we employ the CTX needle with O-Vicryl® suture. The need for vascular suturing during urologic laparoscopy is rare, and is usually done on an emergent basis. Considerable laparoscopic experience is required to perform emergent vascular suturing for hemostasis. In such circumstances, we have preferred the CT-1 needle with 2–0 Vicryl® to control the site of hemorrhage from the vena cava expeditiously.

What Are Your Tips for Laparoscopic Surgery in Obese Patients?

Dr. Gill

The patient should be clearly informed that his/her chances of open conversion are somewhat higher than a normal patients. Also, have extra-long morbid obesity laparoscopic instruments available. Place as many ports as are necessary to do the procedure safely. Finally, it is very important to maintain anatomic orientation along clear anatomic planes. As long as proper orientation is maintained, the operation can be performed safely despite the *volume of fat*. We have had good success with the retroperitoneal approach to renal surgery in the obese patient.

Dr. Stoller

We use the hook cautery very frequently for dissection and I did not realize that there were different lengths of the hook cautery available. I think that different lengths for the hook cautery are critical, especially for obese patients.

Dr. Albala

For nephrectomy work, I have found that moving the trocars off the midline in obese patients toward the kidney allows the renal dissection to be done more easily. If a hand-assisted procedure is being done on a very obese patient, the hand incision needs to be closed in an interrupted fashion. We have had one dehiscence and one hernia that developed when we did a running closure. I think that closing the incision in an interrupted fashion in an obese patient is extremely important. In addition, all our obese patients wear an abdominal binder for one month postoperatively. We feel this places less stress on the incision site and allows for better healing. This is commonly done by our general surgery colleagues when they operate on obese patients. A midline incision tends to be a little stronger than a paramedian incision and these are always closed in an interrupted fashion.

Do You Have General Tips for the Residents?

Dr. Rassweiler

When I work on the prostate, usually I handle the bipolar diathermy with the left hand, and the scissors with the right. I am not a "hook-man," like others! For me the main instruments are the bipolar dissector, scissors, and the right-angle dissector. I only seldom use the peanut dissector. My principle in surgery is to cut whenever you can; and laparoscopy allows you to see very nicely where you can cut. When one does blunt dissection, one doesn't know exactly where one is. Of course, around vessels you may use (the peanut for blunt dissection), but I very much like to use the suction device as a blunt instrument for dissection. So there are only a few cases where I think that the peanut is really helpful. It was different in the beginning, but I must say now with increasing experience I prefer to cut wherever I can.

For renal surgery it is similar but you cannot use bipolar diathermy like prostatectomy because usually it is a three-port technique. So, though I prefer the bipolar diathermy, we do not use it in kidney surgery, because if you do, then you have to switch over to the scissors just to cut after you coagulate something. I tell this to my residents, because they see us operating on the prostate and then try to do the same in renal surgery.

One problem is changing your field too often. What I prefer is for the left hand to retract while the right hand acts. For the sake of time management, the left hand is kept stable while the right hand is active. For example, incise with the right hand; do bipolar coagulation (with the left hand) and incision again with the right hand. What one has to learn from the beginning is the "one hand feeds the other technique." Whatever you do, keep the image still. And then one hand feeds the other.

One more point is that there should not be too much emphasis on keeping the three-trocar setup. The addition of a fourth trocar is usually not a problem. One could use a 3-mm trocar if necessary, but a 5-mm trocar also does not hurt much more. So you should insert an additional port whenever you feel you are not comfortable with the exposure. I think this is very important.

Dr. Lou Kavoussi

Beginners in laparoscopy are tense and tend to raise the table high, as in open surgery. Actually, it is better to drop the table lower because that brings your elbows in, increasing operator comfort. If the elbows are positioned high up, then one is using one's back and shoulder muscles to hold the arms up, which reduces precision. It is much more comfortable operating with the elbows tucked at the side and just using the forearms and wrists. This is the most common mistake that residents and fellows do when beginning to operate; they do a sort of "chicken stance" with their elbows out. One should lower the table and keep the elbows in.

References

1. Khaira, H.S., Wolf, J.S., Jr.: Intraoperative local anesthesia decreases postoperative parenteral opioid requirements for transperitoneal laparoscopic renal and adrenal surgery: A randomized, double-blind, placebo controlled investigation. J Urol **172:** 1422, 2004
2. Landman, J., Venkatesh, R., Kibel, A., et al.: Modified renal morcellation for renal cell carcinoma: Laboratory experience and early clinical application. Urology **62:** 632, 2003

Chapter 2
Simple Nephrectomy

Please Give Three Tips for Laparoscopic Simple Nephrectomy

Dr. de la Rosette

People tend to put in a minimum number of ports for simple nephrectomy, say, three ports, maybe because it's sexy! Maybe you can even do it with two, but I think, when doing simple nephrectomy, one should not be afraid to put in an extra port, if you think that would help and you should not wait too long to do that. From the beginning, if you feel you have chosen the wrong port and need an additional port, just go ahead and put one

in. The second tip is that when you go for the transperitoneal approach you often go for a zero-degree lens, but
if you go in a retroperitoneal approach you absolutely
need the 30-degree lens, because otherwise you will not
have the optimal view. The third tip is that instead of
using a GIA to control the renal vessels you can use the
very nice Wecklock® clip. They are cheap, they are reliable, and they are easy to handle.

Dr. Keeley

A common problem among novices is that they make a
great effort to find the ureter before touching the kidney
and oftentimes find themselves going through a lot of fat
in the retroperitoneum, unable to find the ureter for
quite some time. A very simple technique is first to identify and then lift the lower pole of the kidney, putting it
on stretch and thereby exposing the space medial to it
(Figure 2.1). In doing so, you can lift the ureter and the
hilum away from the colon and the great vessels, so that
further dissection is much easier. If you try to find the
ureter in its native bed or where it usually lies, you find
yourself going through an awful lot of tissue in order to
identify a very small structure. By lifting the lower pole
of the kidney, this brings it much more on stretch.
This is a technique that I learned from David Tolley in
Edinburgh and he in turn learned it from a Russian urologist who was working with Dr. Gerhard Fuchs at UCLA
many years ago in the early 90s. It is nothing new, but
again it is the most common obstacle people come up
against and, I think, oftentimes, people are incorrectly
taught to find the ureter first and put that up on stretch.

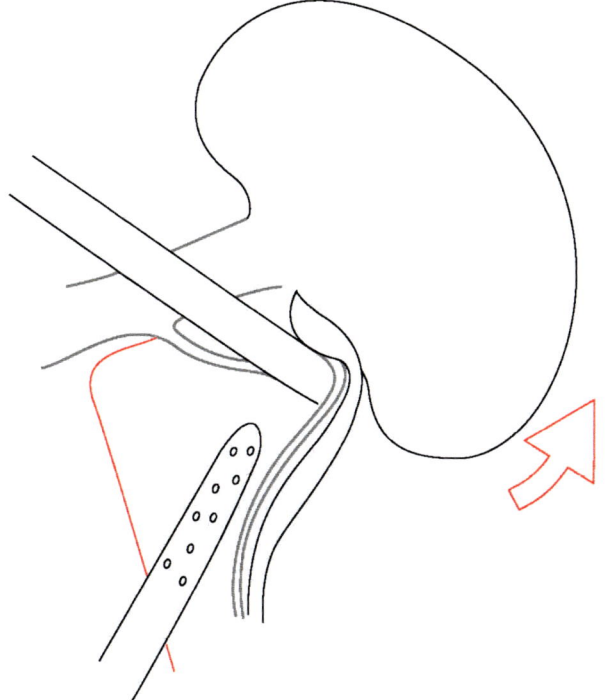

Fig. 2.1 Elevation of lower pole of the kidney.

Another simple technique, which is again nothing new or unusual, is to leave the ureter intact during the dissection, so that you don't have to spend a grasper or a retractor on the cut end of the ureter during a nephrectomy. I've seen people deliberately divide the ureter and then use that as a lever. However, if you leave the ureter intact, you can then use simple blunt instruments to lift the ureter and so the hilum can be put on stretch. This also prevents a common problem at the end of the nephrectomy, which is loss of orientation and twisting of the kidney.

How Does One Find the Renal Hilum During Transperitoneal Laparoscopic Nephrectomy?

Dr. Gill

After reflecting the bowel medially, the ureter and gonadal veins are identified, retracted laterally, and the psoas muscle identified between the ipsilateral great vessel medially and the ureter/gonadal vein laterally. On the left side, the gonadal vein is then traced cephalad to identify the renal vein. At this point, the ureter and gonadal vein are transected en-block in the vicinity of the lower pole of the kidney using an Endo-GIA stapler. The proximal end of the transected ureter and gonadal vein are tightly grasped with locking forceps and retracted antero-laterally, thereby torquing the lower pole of the kidney, upward and outward (Figure 2.2). This will swing the posteriorly located renal artery some-what inferiorly and anteriorly, bringing it into easier view behind the renal vein. Following the gonadal vein cephalad is the best way to identify the left renal vein. We typically place one clip on the renal artery to occlude arterial inflow to the kidney. Thereafter, the renal vein is taken with an Endo-GIA stapler and the renal artery is now clearly visualized and dissected, and additional clips are placed and transected. On the right side, the gonadal vein enters the vena cava and can be clipped and divided to prevent inadvertent injury. As on the left side, the ureter and peri-ureteral fat are transected with an Endo-GIA stapler near the lower pole of the kidney, then grasped and retracted anterolaterally, thereby bringing

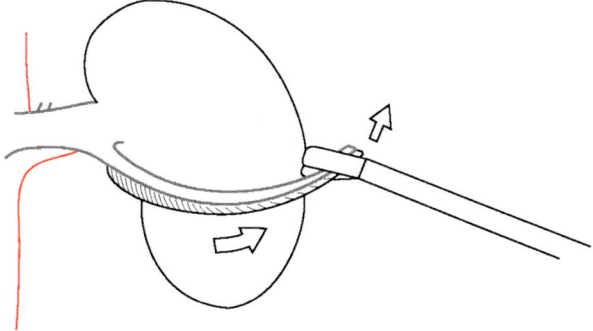

Fig. 2.2 Retraction of the ureter and gonadal vein.

the posteriorly located renal artery into somewhat better view. This is then clipped and occluded. The renal vein is then taken as on the left side, and finally the renal artery is secured.

How to Expose the Renal Artery and Adrenal Vein

Dr. Keeley

In left-sided transperitoneal nephrectomy, one can have difficulty identifying the renal artery because it is lying either right behind or slightly superior to the renal vein. In this situation, the gonadal vein is clipped and transected at some distance from the renal vein. The gonadal vein stump can then be used as a handle to reflect the left renal vein in order to expose the renal artery.

Trying to expose the upper pole of the left kidney or finding the left adrenal transperitoneally, I find, is often times challenging. It is helpful to dissect the peritoneal reflexion lateral to the spleen. Developing the space between the upper pole of kidney and the spleen can allow the spleen to fall more medially and get out of your way, and it will take with it the tail of the pancreas, so that you get to the left adrenal and upper pole of the kidney easier.

Locating the Renal Artery in Retroperitoneal Surgery

Dr. Wolf

In many retroperitoneoscopic cases the artery is obvious once the kidney is lifted up, but in others—usually obese men—the landmarks are indistinct and the location of the artery cannot be determined in the usual fashion (looking for pulsations). We have realized that it is almost always right in front of the port at the base of the 12th rib, or at most a centimeter or two cephalad to this (Figure 2.3). This is an amazingly consistent relationship, and if you are lost it can help you get started every single time!

Dr. Gill

After port placement, the first step is to place the Gerota's fascia-covered kidney on significant lateral traction with a laparoscopic retractor in the surgeon's non-dominant hand. Using a suction or J-hook electrocautery, gentle

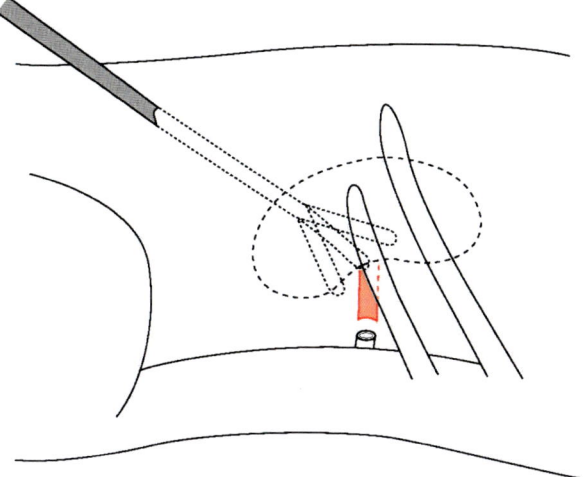

Fig. 2.3 Locating the renal artery.

dissection is performed along the anterior surface of the psoas muscle toward the superomedial direction. At this point, it is important to keep the dissection in the flimsy white fibro-areolar tissue along the ipsilateral great vessel. One must stay anterior to the ipsilateral great vessel, taking care not to stray posterior to it. If dissection is proceeding in the yellow peri-renal fat, one is probably dissecting too close to the renal parenchyma. Again, good lateral counter-traction is important to place the renal hilum on stretch. In general, the renal hilum is located at an angle of 45 to 60 degrees from the vertical. This is the angle that the shafts of your instruments outside the patient's body will be describing when you find the renal vessels. The renal artery is posterior, and the renal vein is anterior and usually caudal (inferior) to the renal artery. Before beginning dissection on the renal artery or vein, the horizontal positions of the major vessels (aorta on the left side, vena cava on the right: both parallel to the psoas) and vertical pulsations of the fat-covered renal artery laterally are looked for, and almost always visualized. We typically control the renal artery with Weck® clips (two toward the aorta, one toward the kidney), and control the renal vein with an Endo-GIA stapler. One must remember that during renal retroperitoneoscopy the psoas is the constant anatomic landmark: the psoas "is your best friend."

Chapter 3
Donor Nephrectomy and Autotransplantation

What Radiographic Imaging is Necessary Before Considering a Patient for Laparoscopic Donor Nephrectomy for Transplantation?

Dr. Gill

In earlier days, conventional arteriography was the standard procedure performed in every patient undergoing a donor nephrectomy. With advances in CT scanning techniques, currently we perform a 3D-CT scan with a video reconstruction as the only preoperative radiographic imaging. The 3D-CT scan provides superb visualization of the renal artery, renal vein, and the interrelationship of these extra-renal vessels. Further, it also evaluates the renal parenchyma for any abnormalities. Finally, the collecting system is imaged as well. I believe that the 3D-CT is the best test for renal vein anatomy. Currently, interventional angiography is performed in addition only in those patients who have multiple renal vessels on 3D-CT. In a recent study, in which 50 potential kidney donors underwent both the 3D-CT scan and conventional arteriography, in every patient that the 3D-CT confirmed a single renal artery and single renal vein bilaterally, arteriography confirmed these findings.[1] However, if a patient had more than one renal artery, which occurred in a small percentage of patients, the arteriogram could potentially identify the additional vessel that has been missed by the 3D-CT. The 3D-CT can also assess the branching distance from the aortic origin of the renal artery on either side. As such, even if there is a single vessel, if the branching distance is short (say, less than 1.5 cm) it is likely that after clipping and dividing the renal artery, the transplant recipient surgeon may be faced with two renal arteries, given that the common stem has been involved in the clipping on the donor. This additional information about branching distance is another anatomic data point that is provided by the 3D-CT, which allows one to select between the left and right kidney.

What Are Your Tips for Performing Donor Nephrectomy?

Dr. Gill

1. To identify the left renal vein, we typically follow the gonadal vein cephalad. The gonadal vein is transected at a reasonable distance of 3 to 4 cm from the renal vein and the cut end of the gonadal vein is then used as an atraumatic handle to manipulate the renal vein during the remainder of the operation.
2. The renal artery is almost always identifiable along the inferior edge of the renal vein. Certainly, the renal vein needs to be completely mobilized in order to *identify the renal artery accurately*. Trying to identify the renal artery cephalad to the renal vein is more difficult and also more dangerous.
3. The renal artery needs to be mobilized only in its proximal 2 cm at the aortic take-off. Further mobilization of the renal artery into the renal hilum is unnecessary, causes vasospasm, and is potentially dangerous.

4. The ureter and gonadal veins should be mobilized as a single packet, with dissection proceeding medial to the gonadal vein. Electrocautery should be applied sparingly in this dissection and the ureter is typically transected at the level of the iliac vessels.

Dr. Jihad Kaouk

1. During left donor nephrectomy, the main renal vein is dissected toward the interaorto-caval area to maximize the length of the harvested renal vein. An Endo-GIA stapler is used to occlude and transect the renal vein. Intentionally, the renal vein is only partially stapled (Figure 3.1) (two thirds of total width) for three reasons: (1) If the Endo-GIA malfunctions, the attached part of the renal vein will avoid complete retraction of the transected left renal vein into the inter aorto-caval area. (2) The superior mesenteric artery is in close proximity to the upper edge of the left renal vein. Chances of Endo-GIA injury to the superior mesenteric artery are minimized by placing the Endo-GIA only across partial circumference of the renal vein. (3) The intact unstapled third of the left renal vein is clipped with Hem-O-Lok® clips toward the vena cava side and then cut with an Endoshears, thus venting the entrapped blood from the kidney.

2. We do not heparinize our laparoscopic donors.

3. Do not cut the ureter before the transplant team examines the recipient vessels and confirms transplantable conditions.

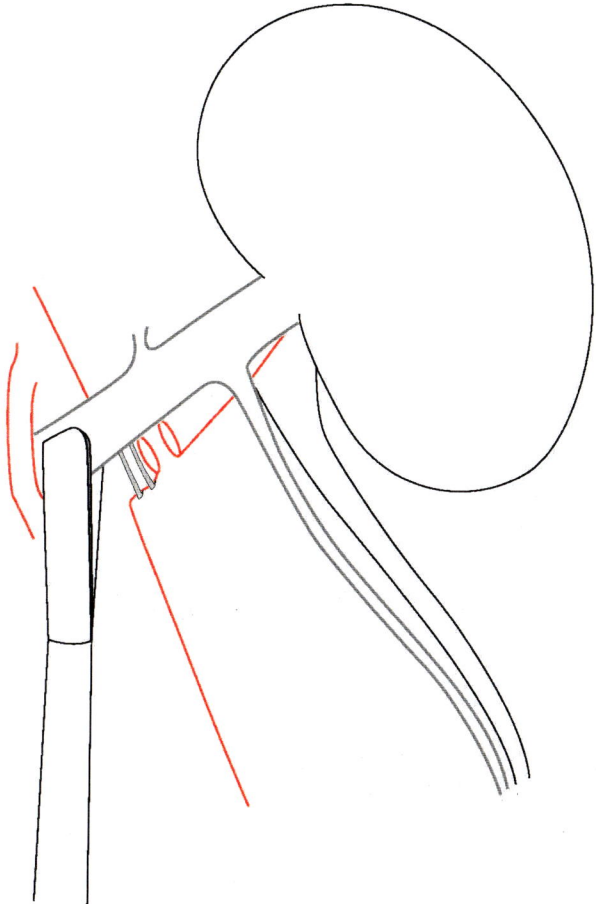

Fig. 3.1 Transection of the left renal vein.

4. The left renal artery is clipped adjacent to the aorta only. The kidney side of the renal artery is not clipped to avoid further loss of the renal artery length. Even in case of multiple renal arteries, retrograde bleeding is not significant enough to compromise surgical exposure.

Dr. Stoller

To dissect the renal artery adequately for a donor nephrectomy, you must dissect the renal artery until you see a "fanning out" or a cone as it originates from the aorta. Failure to identify that expanding cone means that you've not gone all the way to the aorta. For a right-sided donor nephrectomy, there is no need to put any kind of clip on the renal side of the artery. We will use one Weck® clip right next to the aorta and then a titanium clip proximal to that. For the vein we routinely use a TA stapler that just lays three rows of staples with no cutting. Cutting is then performed with laparoscopic scissors. There are no staples on the renal side. That will optimize the length of the renal vein and will ease the transplant when you take the donation from the right side. The TA stapler is very useful. It separates ligation from transection. It also avoids the potential misfires of the GIA stapler.

How Do You Handle a Retro-aortic or Circumaortic Renal Vein during a Left Donor Nephrectomy?

Dr. Gill

Preparation of a left retro-aortic vein is not much different from that of a normal left renal vein. Essentially, the vein is dissected up to the left lateral border of the aorta where it is transected (Figure 3.2). Typically, for a normal left renal vein, we dissect up to the right lateral border of the aorta in the interaorto-caval region and transect the left renal vein at that location. With a circumaortic vein, in our experience, the retro-aortic component of the vein is almost always smaller in diameter than the antero-aortic component. As such, management of the retro-aortic portion of a circumaortic renal vein is essentially similar to that of a large lumbar vein arising from the left renal vein. It is transected between Hem-O-Lok® clips.

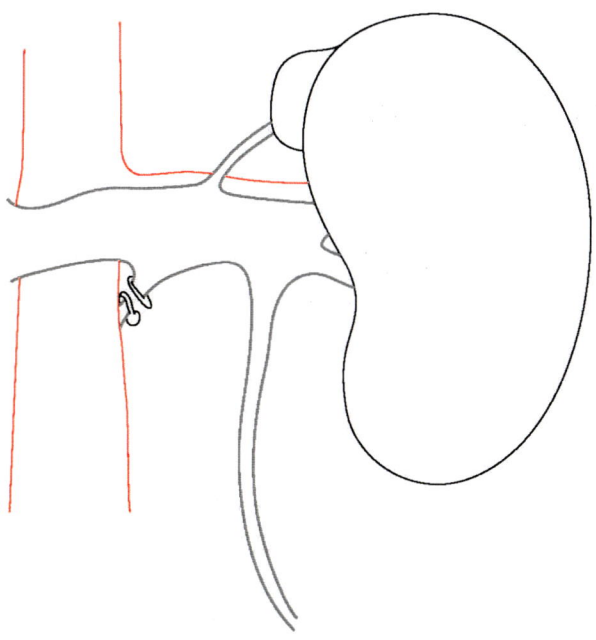

Fig. 3.2 Circum-aortic left renal vein.

Does Laparoscopy Have a Role in Renal Autotransplantation?

Dr. Stoller

For difficult ureteral strictures, laparoscopic reconstructive techniques may work out very well. A spiral flap may sometimes bridge the gap. Unfortunately we are seeing more iatrogenic ureteral injuries where there are large defects up to 15 cm. Traditionally, some people have used ileal interposition to replace the ureter. I personally don't like ileal replacement because of mucous secretions and dilation that can contribute not only to infection but also obstruction and stones. Auto-transplantation is usually performed as a last-ditch effort only in situations where there is a solitary kidney. I think auto-transplantation is a viable option in these cases.

Surgically, we treat patients intraoperatively the same as with a donor nephrectomy, using adequate hydration, intravenous mannitol, and a prepared slush solution to irrigate once the kidney has been removed, just as you would do for a normal renal transplant.

One advantage of doing the nephrectomy portion of the auto-transplant laparoscopically is that you minimize the amount of postoperative pain. Sometimes the nephrectomy is very difficult because of adherent scar tissue, but the beauty is that you can do the auto-transplant nephrectomy laparoscopically and perform the final dissection ex vivo. Occasionally you need to take the renal artery and vein en bloc with a GIA stapler. You may also mobilize the ureter laparoscopically to identify what needs to be done and determine whether you should anastomose the renal pelvis into the native ureter or anastomose the pelvis directly to the bladder.

We've also used auto-transplant in very difficult situations for centrally located renal tumors. If you have a very central tumor and you don't think you can deal with it using laparoscopic or open techniques in situ, you can remove the kidney and perform ex vivo bench surgery, reconstruct, and then auto-transplant.

The last indication would be for a patient with recurrent stone disease in which stone fragments have to pass through a strictured ureter. You could anastomose the renal pelvis directly to the urinary bladder, allowing easier stone passage. We are finding increasing indications for auto-transplantation, and laparoscopic techniques avoid the traditional painful upper abdominal incision for removing the kidney.

Reference

1. El Fettouh, H.A., Herts, B.R., Nimeh, T., et al.: Prospective comparison of 3-dimensional volume rendered computerized tomography and conventional renal arteriography for surgical planning in patients undergoing laparoscopic donor nephrectomy. J Urol **170:** 57, 2003

Chapter 4
Hand-Assisted Laparoscopy

What Is Your Technique for Placement of the Hand-Assistance Device?

Dr. Wolf

Placement of the hand-assistance device depends on the device being used. As opposed to the original hand-assistance devices, the current ones are placed before creating the pneumoperitoneum. The manufacturer's instructions are usually pretty clear, and they should be followed carefully. If you are cavalier about it and don't learn the specifics for insertion of each device, you will struggle a lot. There are particular tricks for applying each individual device. For the Lap Disc®, placing two stay sutures helps considerably. For the Gelport®, rolling the wound protector edge to the right distance and getting the first "snap" of the cap on firmly are important. For the Omniport®, it is easier to place both rings into the abdomen, and then pull the outer one out, than it is to place the inner one inside the abdomen and the outer one outside initially.

In terms of where to place the device, there are many opinions. We still use a vertical midline incision in most cases. A midline incision is easy to open and close, and can be moved cephalad or caudad as desired (Figure 4.1). A problem with this incision, however, is the wound complication rate.[1] Upon retrospective evaluation of 424 consecutive procedures performed at our institution, we found complications at the hand-assistance incision site in 44 patients (10.4%), including 29 infections (6.8%), 15 hernias (3.5%), and 2 dehiscences (0.5%) (2 patients had both infection and hernia). Aside from the 2 dehiscences, the 15 hernias all presented more than three months after surgery—which suggests a wound-healing defect rather than a technical problem with closure. A very nice meta-analysis of prospective or matched retrospective studies of incision placement for general surgery found that the risk of herniation was 8.4% and 5.1% for vertical and transverse incisions, respectively.[2] So perhaps the urologists who place their incision for the hand-assistance device in oblique lower-quadrant incisions

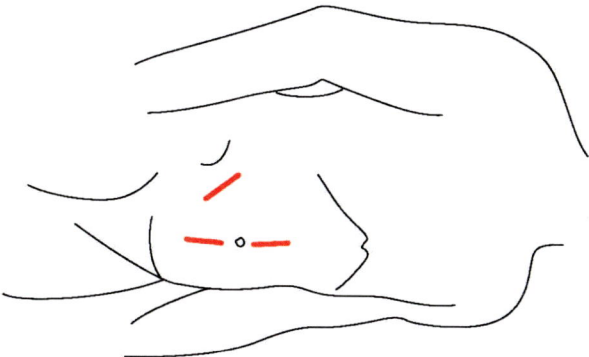

Fig. 4.1 Positions for hand-assistance device placement.

have the right idea. On occasion we have used a transverse Pfannenstiel-type incision. It is a bit more cephalad   than   a   true   Pfannenstiel   incision,   but   the
combination of the transverse anterior fascial incision
and the splitting of the muscle bellies of the rectus abdominis muscle is a less painful incision and may be less
likely to herniate. That remains to be seen.

With regard to port placement in association with
hand-assisted laparoscopic surgery, my tip would be to
use manual guidance instead of inflating and looking in
with the laparoscope. If you are using non-bladed trocars
for your ports, and this technique can only be done with
non-bladed trocars, then you can put your hand through
the hand-assistance site, feel the kidney to determine its
location, decide where to place your ports, manually
make an incision right on top of your fingers, and put
the trocar down right on top of your fingers (Figure 4.2).
It is a much faster way of putting it the ports, probably
cutting ten minutes off the surgical time.

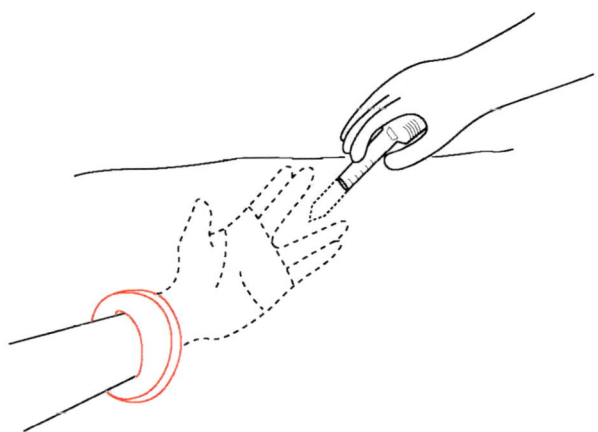

Fig. 4.2 Bimanual placement of ports.

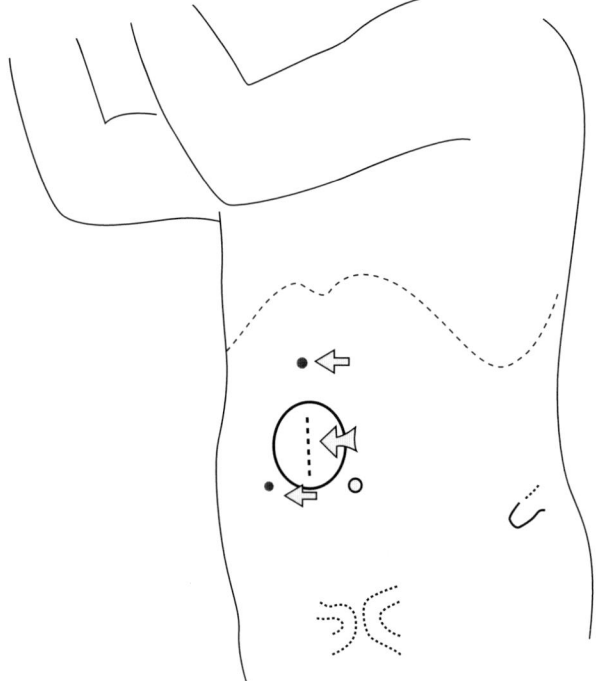

Fig. 4.3 Port placement in obese patients.

Finally, for obese patients, the hand-assistance device in the midline is just too far away from the kidney. The hand-assistance device and the ports are moved cephalad and lateral. Placement of the hand-assistance device through a paramedian incision might be required (Figure 4.3).

Dr. Albala

A variety of locations on the abdomen can be used for the hand-assistance device. On the right side, I like to make a modified Gibson-like muscle splitting incision. For a right-handed surgeon, this will give excellent access to the kidney. On the left side, for the beginner, I found that making an incision around the umbilicus or just above the umbilicus works very nicely. As one gets more experienced, one might consider using an incision below the umbilicus as I think that this gives patients less pain. This position may be difficult for the novice laparoscopic surgeon as it is somewhat of a long reach to get up to the upper pole of the left kidney by the spleen. That is why for the novice laparoscopic surgeon, I typically tell them to make an incision that goes around the umbilicus, extending just above and below the umbilicus, to allow adequate access for the superior aspect of the kidney. For a hand-assisted laparoscopic nephroureterectomy, I like to make an incision starting below the umbilicus and extending downward toward the pubic bone. That seems to work very well, especially when it comes to the dissection of the distal ureter and bladder cuff. Again, this may cause the surgeon to reach to get up to the upper pole of the kidney but the incision is in excellent position for the distal ureter and bladder cuff.

What Hand Port Device Do You Prefer and Why?

Dr. Stephen Nakada

I generally prefer the Gelport (Applied Medical, Santa Margarita, CA), and the main reason is that it maintains the pneumoperitoneum when you exchange hands. As we train residents, we will alternate the surgeon and you can do this and retain the pneumoperitoneum. This is also very useful during a partial nephrectomy and it is also gives you the option of placing another instrument through the device. At this time the Gelport is the most versatile device, but it is more expensive than other devices and it is a little more complex to set up. So I recommend the Gelport, although the Omni Port and Lap Disc are effective for many people.

How You Prevent Hand Fatigue?

Dr. Nakada

Well, I think the real misnomer in hand-assisted laparoscopy is that you perform most of the dissection with your hand. I think, if you have hand fatigue, you're probably overutilizing your hand to dissect. We utilize the hand to pick up tissue and help set up the field, and the majority of the procedure is still done with a laparoscopic instrument, and so if your hand is getting tired you probably need to work on your port placement and trocar location.

Any Tips for Port Placement?

Dr. Nakada

One nice thing with hand-assisted laparoscopy is that, sometimes in a challenging abdomen, you can make the hand incision first. So you can make the 7-cm incision and then eliminate the risk of the Veress needle and the complexity of Hasson cannula access. On the other hand, you may not always know where you are going to put the hand-assist device and if you make the incision first, you have to use it. So my approach for many hand-assisted cases is to use the Veress needle, get in an initial trocar, look around, and then decide where I am going to put the hand port and my trocars. Really, it probably is very hard to have one template for port placement, just because each patient and pathology is different. But generally, the goal is to have your non-dominant hand be in the abdomen. Usually for a right-handed person, for a left-sided nephrectomy the incision is lower umbilical. For a right nephrectomy the incision is going to be a sub costal muscle splitting incision.

What Sort of Hand Incision Do You Use for Nephroureterectomy: i.e., Right Versus Left?

Dr. Nakada

That is a good question. Generally, on the right you definitely are going to use a MacBurney's incision and on the left, probably go lower midline, because I think you like having an option of doing the bladder cuff open. Generally, I believe that with a nephroureterectomy, if there is no ureteral tumor, I definitely favor doing an extensive dissection to the bladder, stapling the bladder cuff, and then cystoscopically unroofing the ureteral orifice.

On the Left Side if You Place the Hand Incision Sub-Umbilical, Occasionally It Is Hard to Reach the Kidney through That Incision or the Lower Incision Makes the Hand Fatigue a Bit More. Do You Have Any Tips to Overcome That?

Dr. Nakada

Generally it is tricky if you have a short arm and you have a tall patient, but usually one thing that is helpful is, in the obese patient, you should go lateral to midline: moving your trocars off midline will make a difference because the kidney, if you are doing a transperitoneal approach, is certainly going to be fairly posterior and you don't want to be too far from the target organ. By the same token if you are doing a left nephroureterectomy, I think you should try to make your incision such that you can do the nephrectomy first and worry more about the bladder cuff later.

How Does One Use the Hand for Maximum Impact During Hand Assistance?

Dr. Wolf

Optimal use of the hand during hand-assisted laparoscopic surgery requires that you use your wrist and fingers in many bizarre sorts of ways. Don't constrain yourself to using your hands like they are used during open surgery. You need to make odd combinations of positions with your wrists and your fingers: extending the wrist while flexing the fingers, twisting the hand and extending a thumb, lifting one structure up and away while palpating with a different finger, etc. Use your hand in as many multi-functional positions as possible—that is my number one tip.

The second thing to remember is that the hand is a good exploring instrument, it is a good retracting instrument, and it is a good exposing instrument—but its use as a dissecting instrument should be limited. Surgeons first using hand assistance tend to use the hand too much for dissecting; this tires the hand more quickly and risks bleeding and tissue injury. Some gross dissection is fine, but delicate dissection should not be done bluntly by the intra-abdominal hand. A useful multifunctional maneuver for hand-assisted laparoscopic kidney surgery, dubbed the C-position by Dr. Steven Strup, is to flex the wrist, elevate the lower pole with the index finger, provide tension on medial tissues with the thumb, hold back bowel with the back of the hand and wrist, and carefully explore the renal hilum with the middle finger (Figure 4.4). To gain control of the hilum, dissect the inferior and anterior aspects of the hilum sharply, elevating the lower pole of the kidney with an assisting instrument (freeing up the index finger in the process), and then sneak that finger superiorly around the hilum with the goal of encircling the hilar vessels between the index finger and the thumb (Figure 4.5). This is one good use of the hand for blunt dissection, but only if it goes very easily. If it does not, then you stop. Again, many

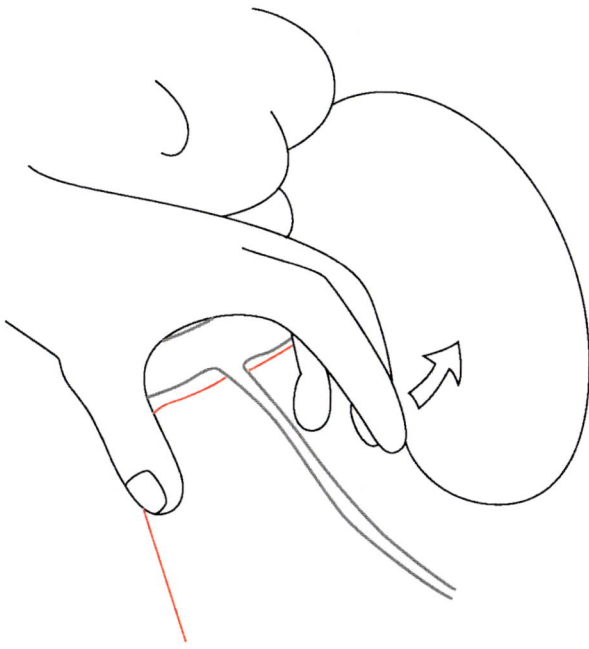

Fig. 4.4 The "C-position".

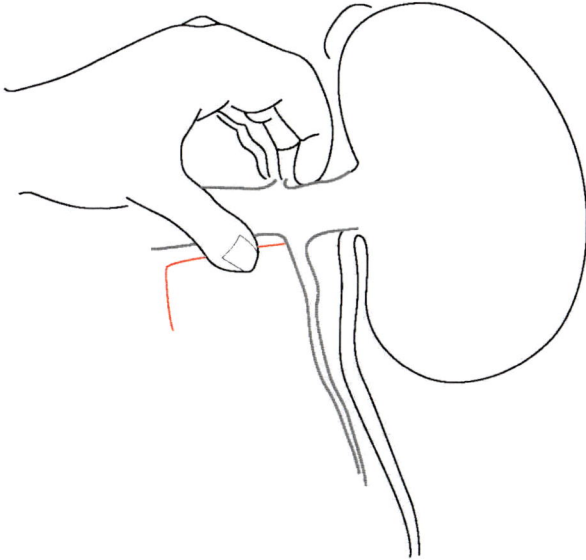

Fig. 4.5 Encircling the hilum.

novices will persist too long in dissecting with the hand and it gets them into trouble. Most of the dissection still should be performed with instruments.

How Does One Keep the Hand out of the Way During Hand-Assisted Laparoscopic Surgery?

Dr. Albala

The most important point when doing hand-assisted laparoscopic surgery is to insure that you have an adequate pneumoperitoneum. Typically, when performing this type of surgery, the hand doesn't block the camera view. A blocked view occurs when the abdominal pressure decreases and the hand occupies all the free space in the abdomen. This most commonly occurs when you are doing a hand-assisted left nephrectomy. In this situation, one trocar site is in the midline and the other trocar site is in the midclavicluar line. I sometimes will switch my hands and put my dominant hand into the abdominal cavity to do some of the dissection. When I place my right hand in the abdomen on the left side, an unobstructed view of the abdominal contents usually results. I found that if you can be somewhat ambidextrous and allow the dissection to be accomplished with both hands, the cases go much easier. The second point to insure an unobstructed view is to place the initial trocars to allow maximum visualization. For example, if the patient is very obese, I tend to place my trocars off the midline and more toward the side of the tumor. This allows for an unobstructed view and it also makes the dissection easier. If the tumor is very large, there isn't really a good method to keep your hand from obstructing the camera because of the limited space.

Can One Combine the Advantages of Standard Laparoscopic and Hand-Assisted Laparoscopic Surgery?

Dr. Kumar

Ponsky and associates advise placing the hand-assist device in the right- or left-lower quadrant using a Gibson muscle-splitting incision.[3] They place a trocar through the hand-access device and perform traditional laparoscopy, alternating this with use of the intra-abdominal hand for dissection and extraction of the specimen.

How Do You Deal With an Air Leak through Your Hand Port?

Dr. Nakada

Well, if you are leaking from the hand port first, you have to really check to make sure it is inserted correctly. The other possibility is that often in obese patients, it is difficult to get the device seated properly due to the extended distance the device must traverse. I think the good news is that today the hand devices are very effective. Generally, leaks are a thing of the past, at least in my view. I think the big problem with leaks originally was that any device that you glued on became problematic. Occasionally, we will use a wet lap sponge around the base of the device, or tighten the incision using a towel clip. Sometimes a new device is necessary.

Dr. Albala

Whenever there is a gas leak during laparoscopic surgery, you need to check where the gas leak is coming from. Often the gas leak may be from a faulty trocar valve. Initially, I check all the trocar sites and if I find a faulty valve in a trocar, I would replace that trocar with a new one. If that doesn't work and I find out that the leakage is from the hand-assist site, a number of simple maneuvers can be done to stop the leakage. How this problem is corrected may be related to the hand-assisted device being used. With the Applied Medical Gelport® device, typically the leakage comes from around where the inner ring has been placed. In this situation, I will disassemble the whole ring, pull it out of the abdomen, and check it for any puncture holes. If the ring looks fully intact and there's no problem, then the air leakage could be coming from the incision itself. In these cases, the most common problem is that the incision site is too long. I typically address this by placing a Vaseline gauze around that area to try to isolate this space from further gas leakage. In addition, I may also place a towel clip at the skin edges to reduce the leakage. With the Ethicon Lapdisc®, I use similar techniques to stop the gas leakage. This device tends to have a higher gas-leakage rate in my experience. Also, it is much easier to perforate the Lapdisc membrane and if it occurs, a new hand-assist device needs to be used. Whenever I use the Lapdisc, I try to ensure that no sharp objects are placed in the vicinity of this device.

Do You Find Hand Assistance Useful for Intra-Corporeal Suturing?

Dr. Nakada

Yes, for partial nephrectomies. I think one nice thing is that it is very easy to suture (with hand assistance) and I think for many urologists, a hand-assisted partial nephrectomy should include suture repair of the parenchyma for hemostasis and possibly collecting system repair. I think people that do hand-assisted procedures should refine their suturing skills early on because then they can be used both to get out of potential bleeding situations and for performing partial nephrectomies. Essentially similar techniques as in pure laparoscopy apply, only that it is much easier to control the needle and to tie the knot (Figure 4.6).

Dr. Albala

When doing a hand-assisted laparoscopic procedure that requires suturing, I think one has to become facile with the instrumentation. I have found the Ethicon needle driver to be the easiest instrument to use. In order to make suturing easier, one needs to practice outside of the operating room with the needle driver and a

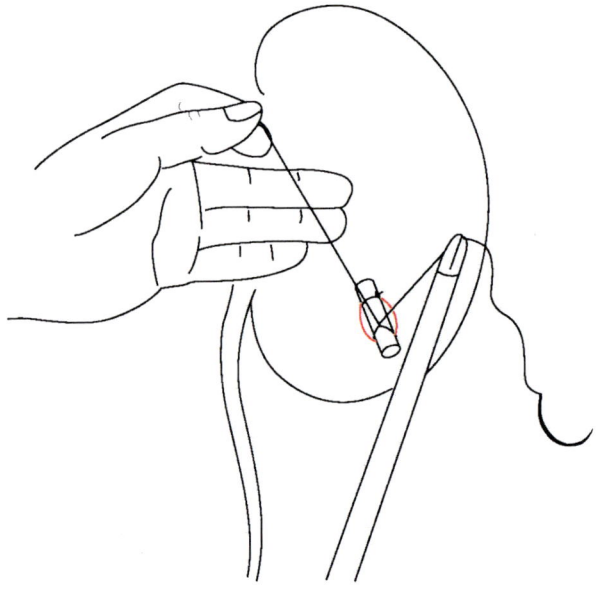

Fig. 4.6 Hand-assisted knot placement.

pelvitrainer. The Lapra-Ty® clip makes things easier, especially during a partial nephrectomy, when one wishes to decrease the warm ischemia time. This device is easy to use and saves a great deal of time. In partial nephrectomy cases, I have found that using a Lapra-Ty® after the suture has been pulled against the bolster works very nicely. In my hands this significantly decreases the warm ischemia time on the kidney.

References

1. Montgomery, J.S., a. W., J.S., Jr.: Wound complications after hand-assisted laparoscopic surgery (HALS). J. Urology **173 supplement:** 317, 2005

2. Grantcharov, T.P., a. R., J.: Vertical compared with transverse incisions in abdominal surgery. European Journal of Surgery **167**: 260, 2001

3. Ponsky, L.E., Cherullo, E.E., Banks, K.L., et al.: Laparoscopic radical nephrectomy: Incorporating advantages of hand assisted and standard laparoscopy. J Urol **169**: 2053, 2003

Chapter 5
Radical Nephrectomy and Nephro-Ureterectomy

What Is Your Essential Technique for Performing Laparoscopic Radical Nephrectomy?

Dr. Christopher Eden

For radical nephrectomy, it is extremely important to get onto the psoas muscle and then develop the plane immediately anterior to it. This leads to the aorta on the left and the IVC on the right. Stay on that great vessel to take the artery first and to take the vein second. You don't always have to do it in that order but if you are going to take the vein first, you need to be prepared for venous hypertension, i.e., bleeding from the venous staple line or from capsular incisions. This is not relevant for radical nephrectomy but can be a problem during a simple nephrectomy of a stone-bearing kidney with a lot of perirenal fibrosis.

Dr. Kaouk

If the main renal artery could not be dissected from behind the main renal vein, then the renal vein is circumferentially dissected and the tissue behind the renal vein (which contains the renal artery) can be stapled using a vascular Endo-GIA. Care should be taken to avoid partial stapling of the renal artery, which can result in hemorrhage.

Excessive flexion of the operating table is not required during the transperitoneal approach and may actually increase the risk of rhabdomyolysis or musculoskeletal postoperative pain.

How about Retroperitoneal Laparoscopic Radical Nephrectomy?

Dr. Kaouk

This is our preferred approach for morbidly obese patients or the occasional pregnant patient undergoing a radical nephrectomy.

The tip of the 12th rib is the main landmark for establishing the initial retroperitoneal access. However, palpating the tip of the 12th rib may be difficult in obese patients. While the patient is in the 90-degree flank position, the ribs should be palpated and marked prior to flexion of the operating table. Using ultrasound or a spinal needle to confirm rib position is helpful. After the skin incision is made at the tip of the 12th rib, the surgeon should reconfirm the rib position by finger palpating the rib through the skin incision before proceeding to incision of the lumbodorsal fascia and entering the retroperitoneal space.

The operative table is flexed just enough to widen the space between the subcostal margin and the iliac crest to insert the retroperitoneal ports. After retroperitoneal ports are inserted, the flexion can be reversed. Again, this will minimize the risk of rhabdomyolysis or musculoskeletal postoperative pain.

Any Tips for Renal Hilar Dissection?

Dr. Stoller

To dissect the hilum, my trick for finding the renal artery on the left side is to follow the gonadal vein to the renal vein. I then use two Aesculap® Prestige graspers (Aesculap, Inc., 3773 Corporate Parkway, Center Valley, PA 18034). The left grasper lifts the vein up and my right grasper does the gentle blunt dissection (Figure 5.1). As long as you stay right behind the vein, there should be nothing behind it except the renal artery, which you can then dissect. Whether you are doing a donor nephrectomy or a radical nephrectomy, this is a very useful technique. We dissect right underneath the vein on top of the aorta because there are lumbar veins communicating with the left renal vein. On the right side, we will go ahead and do the same technique with the right hand

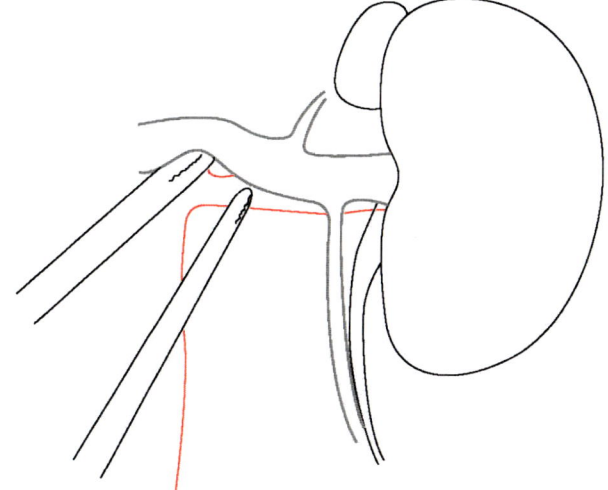

Fig. 5.1 Dissecting the renal artery.

lifting up the renal vein; if you hug right behind the renal vein there's nothing that you're going to get in trouble with and we find that to be an excellent method of accessing the renal artery.

Dr. Kumar

The left gonadal vein is the most important structure to identify during a left nephrectomy as it reliably leads the surgeon to the left renal vein.[1] Retracting the lower pole of the left kidney laterally with an instrument or with the back of the fingers when using hand assistance allows one to place the hilum on stretch, facilitating tracing the course of the gonadal vein and dissection of the renal vein.

Dr. Suzuki

In retroperitoneal laparoscopy, identifying the renal artery is usually straightforward since the artery is most superficial when one dissects along the iliopsoas muscle. One should carefully look for pulsations of the artery.

During transperitoneal surgery, the artery is usually posterior to the renal vein and is often obscured. One tip is to use the 0-degree telescope inserted through the umbilical port to observe for pulsations just posterior to the renal vein.

What Is Your Technique for Hilar Control during Transperitoneal Nephrectomy?

Dr. Kavoussi

On the left side it is important to identify the gonadal vein early. Tracing and dissecting the gonadal vein in a cephalad direction aids in identification of the renal vein. Once the renal vein has been identified, by bluntly dissecting just posterior to the vein, one can create a packet of tissue posteriorly. Typically, there's nothing in the packet other than lymphatic tissue and the renal artery and so one can GIA across that tissue without having to dissect out the artery. When firing the GIA stapler, one must stay quite lateral to the aorta. The advantage to this technique is that one gets less bleeding and obtains rapid control of the arterial blood supply to the kidney. Thereafter, the renal vein can be stapled independently.

On the right side, the renal vein is short and empties directly into the vena cava. Nevertheless, if one identifies the right gonadal vein and stays just lateral to it, the ureter can be found. By tracing the ureter proximally, the renal vein can be identified. Dissecting gently posterior to the vein, hugging right underneath it, and then placing the GIA across the created posterior packet would secure the artery.

Dr. Ono

Originally we used metal clips—three on the aorta side and two clips on the renal side—and divided the artery. We now are using the Hem-O-Lok® clips. They are more reliable. But the Hem-O-Lok clip can injure tissue and you have to ensure to dissect all around the renal artery before placing it. For the renal vein we usually use the Endo-GIA stapler. We have experience in over 500 nephrectomies, including radical and simple nephrectomies and nephroureterectomies, but we have had no problem with malfunction of the stapling device. While some others have reported malfunction of the GIA stapler, that has not happened to us.

Dr. Kumar

If an adequate length of renal artery cannot be dissected free for placement of four or five clips prior to its division, due to its being obscured by the overlying renal vein, one or two clips may be placed across the artery to occlude it. The renal vein may then be safely transected with the Endo-GIA stapler. This allows the renal artery to be visualized for better dissection and division after placement of more clips.

Dr. Kavoussi recommends that sometimes the renal artery can be secured by freeing the anterior, superior, and inferior borders of the renal artery and securing it with the Endo-GIA stapler. In this maneuver, the posterior aspect of the artery is not dissected. However, one must develop the dissection deeply along the superior and inferior borders of the artery until the psoas muscle is clearly visualized, to ensure that the entire width of the artery is included within the jaws of the stapler.[2]

Observe the renal vein after occlusion or division of the renal artery. The vein should collapse with little or no blood flow. If it does not, one should look carefully for additional renal arteries.

If the artery is not clearly visualized from the front (in transperitoneal approach), one may dissect to free the kidney attachments all around and flip the kidney medially and then secure the artery from behind. However, on the right side be wary of injury to the inferior vena cava during this maneuver.

How about En Bloc Division of the Renal Hilum?

Dr. Kumar

In select cases when the renal artery and vein cannot be secured individually, such as severe scarring around the hilum, it is acceptable to secure the renal artery and vein en bloc. An Endo-GIA stapler is used to transect the hilum. In a recent retrospective study, Rapp et al. did not

find any evidence of arterio-venous fistula or other complications following en bloc division of the renal hilum.[3]
The following important steps must be followed when
performing en bloc stapling:

1. The aorta/IVC and the psoas must be in clear
   view
2. The stapler must be fired as close to the kidney
   surface (as far away from the aorta/IVC) as possible
3. Make sure the bowel is retracted out of the way
4. Keep the superior mesenteric artery in mind

While it is recommended that the artery and vein be
secured individually whenever possible, en bloc ligation
can be used safely in select cases. To minimize chances
of arterio-venous fistula formation, one can place multiple 10-mm titanium clips tangentially across the staple
line, thereby effectively clip-occluding any potential A-V
fistula site (Figure 5.2).

Dr. Laguna

The only tip I would like to give is that some times we
use a single firing of the Endo-GIA stapler to take the
entire renal pedicle (artery and vein) en bloc. We have
been doing this without any problems. At the AUA
meeting in 2004, there was a paper that addressed this
issue and they too reported no problems with this
approach. We have not had any arterio-venous fistula
using this approach. The moderator of that session (Dr.
Novick) confirmed the rarity of a fistula in the modern
surgical era.

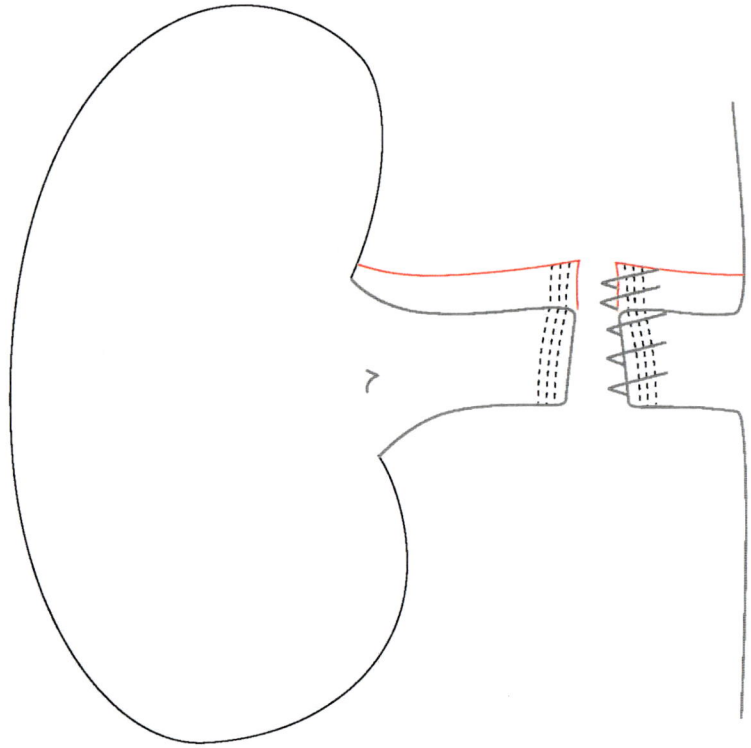

Fig. 5.2 Clips across en-bloc stapled hilum to prevent A-V fistula.

On the Right Side, Do You Take the Renal Artery Behind the Inferior Vena Cava?

Dr. Ono

On the right side, the renal vein is short and identifying the renal artery behind the renal vein during radical nephrectomy may not be easy. So we approach the renal artery from a posterior direction. Our laparoscopic method for radical nephrectomy is to reflect the posterior peritoneum, and then the posterior side of the kidney is dissected off the psoas muscle. The kidney is medially rotated and retracted. This way we expose the artery first and then the vein (Figure 5.3). We do not dissect the anterior aspect of the kidney till we have divided the artery and vein approaching them from behind.

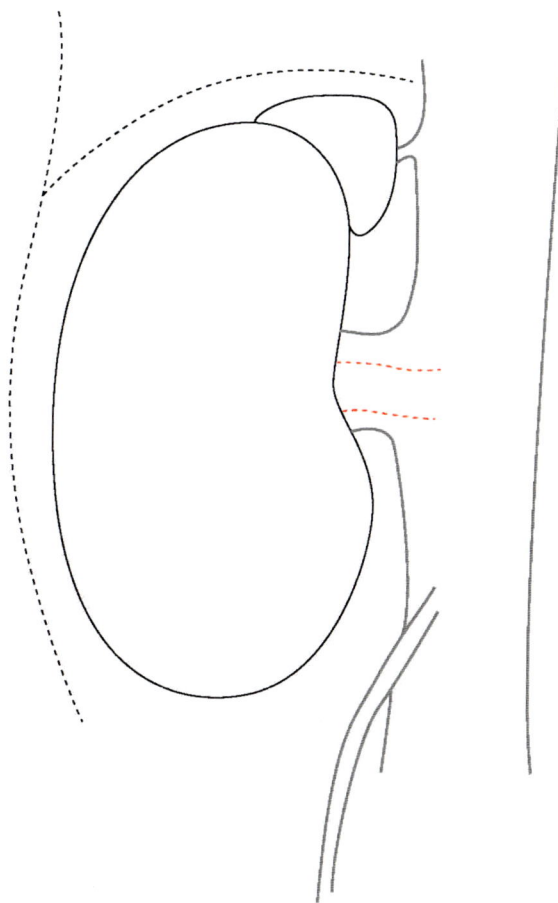

Fig. 5.3 An alternative technique for control of the renal artery.

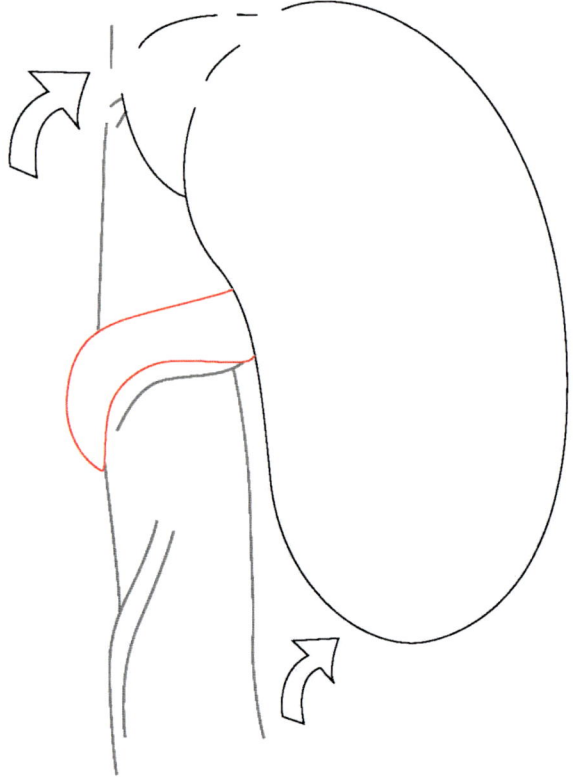

Fig. 5.3 *Continued*

What Are Your Three Tips for Performing Laparoscopic Radical Nephrectomy?

Dr. Cadeddu

The first thing I think about laparoscopic radical nephrectomy is how to handle the hilum. My practice is very similar to the technique used by Lou Kavoussi, MD, at John Hopkins. I would say I almost never dissect out the renal artery and dissect it completely from the renal vein. Rather, the well-described technique by Dr. Kavoussi is my technique: I identify a plane posterior to the renal vein. Then I staple all the tissue behind the renal vein, including the renal artery en mass. I use a GIA stapler for that. I reload the stapler and then just divide the renal vein en mass with its associated tissue that is anterior and superior to it. The posterior wall of the vein has already been identified and so I usually can handle a renal hilum in my opinion very safely and rapidly; and I think that is a big reduction in operative time and an advantage because I don't have to dissect and skeletonize these two vessels. The only time I ever skeletonize the renal artery and vein is when I do donor nephrectomies. I never skeletonize it during laparo-scopic radical nephrectomy.

Another tip for radical nephrectomy: I like to do most nephrectomies using a transperitoneal approach. It is easier to teach and has a larger working volume. I think it is a very important point for the beginner to recognize the plane between the mesentery of the colon and ante-rior Gerota's fascia. It is very important to try and iden-tify that plane so as not to violate the mesentery. Most commonly, beginners will either enter Gerota's fascia because they are too deep or if they are too shallow in the sense they don't recognize the different fat planes and they make perforations in the mesentery. The risk of mesenteric windows is of an internal bowel hernia which is rare but it could happen and it has happened to me. I think a very important tip for beginners is to try to have their mentor re-emphasize that plane and be comfortable recognizing the plane when you are peeling the colon off the anterior aspect of the kidney.

The third thing would be when you do a transperitoneal nephrectomy and after the colon is reflected, I like to identify the ureter and then use that as a landmark that I follow to the renal hilum. Identifying the ureter transperitoneally is another confusing step for beginners. Most of the time one should expect to see the gonadal veins on the anterior surface or just within Gerota's fascia. The first structure therefore that you want to always see is the gonadal vein. If you think you have the ureter and you only have one structure, it is almost always the gonadal vein. Once you identify the gonadal vein, the ureter is posterior and somewhat lateral to the gonadal vein, when the camera is placed in the midline. So when you are looking from the midline at the gonadal vessels, the ureter is posterior and just lateral to the gonadal vessels. So one tip would be, when you think you have the ureter, if you only have one structure, it is most likely the gonadal vessels. Identify them going down to the inguinal ring and then go back and look for the ureter.

How Do You Handle the Bladder Cuff during Laparoscopic Radical Nephroureterectomy?

Dr. Kavoussi

For excising a bladder cuff, we usually do a complete laparoscopic stapling by the extravesical approach. As such, we trace the ureter distally below the iliac vessels up to the bladder. Early on during the dissection we clip the ureter, to avoid spillage of any tumor cells. Then an incision is made in the peritoneum medial to the medial umbilical ligament and the bladder is freed toward the pubic bone. The superior vesical artery pedicle is clipped and divided. This frees the lateral aspect of the bladder and allows the ureter to be followed distally, all the way to its entry point into the bladder. It is important to ensure that one is right on the bladder wall, as there is a lot of thick tissue in the vicinity of the uretero-vesical junction area and one can mistakenly believe that the dissection is more distal than it actually is. One way to ensure this is to continue to tease tissue off and assume that you're not distal enough until you get some bleeding. Upon reaching the detrusor muscle, one sees a little bit more bleeding, whereupon, the stapler can be applied. It is also important to check the foley balloon. The Foley balloon in the bladder is manipulated to ensure that the catheter is not caught in the stapler jaws before it is fired. One should also be careful not to dissect too far across! It helps to have the Foley catheter in the bladder to prevent inadvertent transection of the urethra or the contra-lateral ureter. Importantly, the stapler is inserted from a medial-to-lateral orientation with a postero-lateral tilt to avoid potential injury to the contralateral ureteral orifice. Cystoscopic confirmation at the end of the procedure ensures integrity of the contralateral ureteral orifice, and also confirms that a reasonable cuff of bladder has been excised.

Dr. Keeley

There are many ways described for dealing with the distal ureter and bladder cuff because it can be the most

challenging part of a laparoscopic nephroureterectomy.
The ureter should be clipped in continuity below the
level of the tumor and the ureter dissected down to the
ureterovesical junction. The tip is to start cutting the cuff
of bladder on the superior side of the orifice which of
course is easier when you are approaching it laparoscopically (Figure 5.4). Make sure you can see the Foley
catheter to ensure that you have entered the bladder.
Identify the orifice through the cystotomy in order to
plan the rest of the cuff excision. Before you completely
divide the cuff of bladder, start placing interrupted
sutures in while you have the ureter on stretch, because

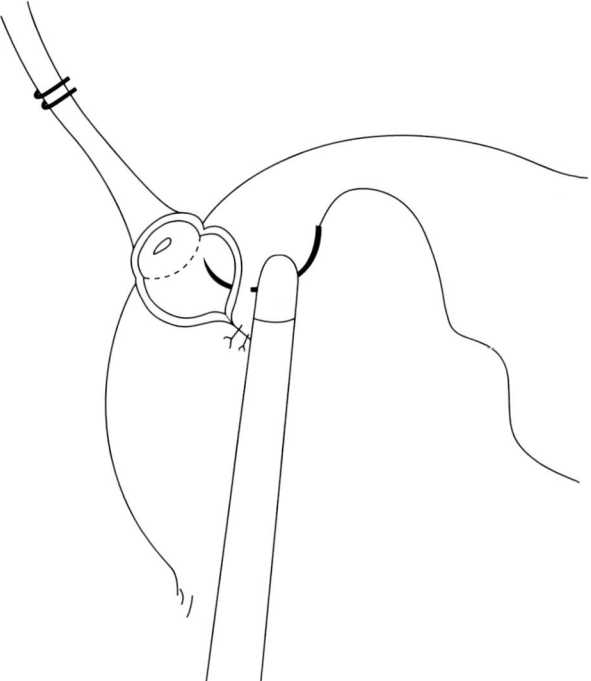

Fig. 5.4 Securing the bladder cuff.

once the ureter is cut, the bladder tends to retract from you and it is difficult to place sutures after that. You can then use some of these as stay sutures. Remember to close the defect before you finish excising the specimen.

How Do You Perform a Lymph Node Dissection during Radical Nephrectomy?

Dr. Ono

Usually the patient positioning is semilateral, 45 to 60 degrees. This is similar to the position for radical nephrectomy. The trocar sites are also similar. With lymph node involvement, dissection can be more difficult because the lymph nodes are often posterior to the vena cava. So we have to transect the lumbar veins to remove the nodes. We have to be careful to avoid injuring the lumbar veins, as these can result in a significant amount of bleeding. Initially on the right side, we dissect the lymph nodes and all the fatty tissue along the vena cava and then we remove the lymph nodes in an en bloc fashion. We then approach the posterior aspect of the vena cava from the bifurcation of the aorta to the renal hilum. While we carefully dissect the posterior aspect of the vena cava, we usually find one or two, sometimes three, lumbar veins. We usually place about three clips on the lumbar veins (the lumbar veins are usually not very long) and divide them (Figure 5.5). We dissect to the level of the renal artery and remove the lymph nodes around the renal artery.

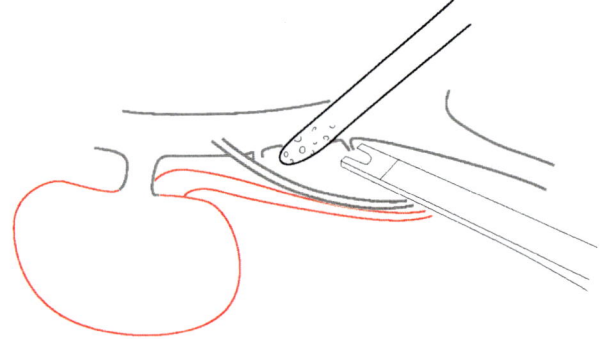

Fig. 5.5 Securing the lumbar veins.

In left-side disease, we usually dissect cranially from the bifurcation of aorta. In about 20% of patients, we find lumbar veins on the left. In some cases near the renal artery, we find lumbar vein branches that may drain into the renal vein. Dissection on the left side is relatively easy if injury of the lumbar vein does not occur. Since we dissect the lymph nodes from the aorta, we can easily identify the renal artery and dissect the lymph nodes from around it also.

How Do You Achieve Retrocaval Clearance for a Retroperitoneal Lymph Node Dissection (RPLND)?

Dr. Kavoussi

It is important to dissect slowly and try to avoid excessive tension because one can very easily disrupt the lumbar veins, leading to troublesome hemorrhage. The vena cava can be held with an atraumatic small bowel clamp or De Bakey-type forceps. If the vena cava is to be grasped, a large purchase should be taken and held steady; taking a small bite could tear the vena cava. One should take a large purchase on the vena cava, lift it anteriorly, and by dissecting posteriorly, the lumbar veins can be clearly displayed, clipped, and divided. Now, if a tear occurs where the lumbar vein drains into the vena cava, it responds nicely to tamponade pressure. Just placing a gauze pad underneath and holding pressure for five to ten minutes usually takes care of such bleeding. Certainly, introducing the hemostatic agent Floseal® onto the site can help significantly in achieving hemostasis in combination with pressure. Depending on one's level of expertise with intracorporeal suturing, one or two attempts at suture control of the venotomy site can be made; we recommend using a CT-1 needle with 2-0 Vicryl for such suturing, which must be done expertly and expeditiously. Continued attempts to over-sew the torn lumbar vein posteriorly may be risky, and one ends up losing a lot more blood, increasing the risk of conversion to open surgery. Likewise, when dissecting posterior to the aorta, one should not actually grasp the aorta because that risks potential injury and plaque fracture in the aorta even though these are usually young patients. So the aorta is elevated by gently leveraging the aorta anteriorly with an atraumatic grasper. This readily allows one to visualize the lumbar arteries. Always leave a 3–4-mm stump on the clipped lumbar artery; one should not divide the lumbar artery too close to the aorta because if the clip slips off of them, then one does not have a stump to re-clamp, and over-sewing is difficult in that location. At all times, the decision to convert to open surgery is available; one must realistically weigh one's personal expertise vis-à-vis the given clinical situation.

Do You Use Any Bipolar Cautery for the Dissection?

Dr. Ono

Usually we prefer ultrasonic scissors made by Olympus. It has better coagulation than the Harmonic scalpel. We also use bipolar electrocautery for hemostasis of small vessels and lymph ducts. An important point is, on the left side, one has to be aware of possible diaphragmatic injury. Close to the trunk of the left renal artery, along the aorta, is the crus of the diaphragm. If the crus is divided, it can result in pneumothorax. In right side dissections, sometimes, interaorto-caval lymph nodes can pose a problem with dissection. Then we have to change the patient position from 60 to 70 degrees lateral to about 40 to 45 degrees and this can make the dissection a little easier.

Any Tips to Control Bleeding from Lumbar Veins during Lymphadenectomy?

Dr. Ono

The lumbar veins can be easily injured close to their entry point into the vena cava. If this happens, do not try to hurry! We usually place a gauze in the working space and in case of bleeding, the assistant tamponades it with the gauze and the suction instrument. We then carefully remove the gauze and identify the bleeding area. If it is from a tear in the lumbar vein, we first clip the distal side, cut the vein and then place two or three clips on the vena caval side across the point of entry of the lumbar vein (Figure 5.6). This usually controls the bleeding.

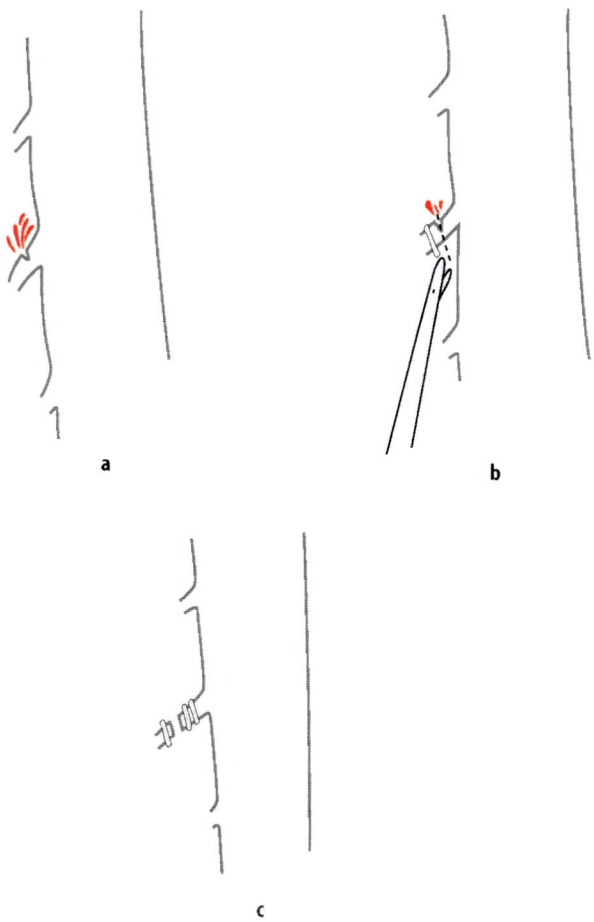

Fig. 5.6 Handling a tear in the lumbar vein.

How Do You Perform Specimen Morcellation?

Dr. Stoller

With morcellation of the kidney or any kind of specimen during laparoscopy, one needs a methodical technique to avoid spillage of any malignant cells. One needs to be careful not to seed the port. We will put three 3 M drapes right next to the port site. We will then put two separate towel drapes. We will then put a half-sheet down. All instruments that we use are considered contaminated and placed on the half sheet. At the end of the morcellation process we will take everything off the field, change gloves and gowns and then proceed with the remainder of the case.

What Are Your Principles of Laparoscopic Radical Nephrectomy for Renal Vein and IVC Involvement?

Dr. Desai

Laparoscopic techniques have been utilized for treating select renal tumors with level I and level II involvement. Appropriate preoperative imaging is critical in this group of patients for optimal surgical planning. We obtain a volume-rendered spiral CT scan with 3D reconstruction in all patients with level I and II venous involvement. While most level I and some early level II

thrombi can be managed laparoscopically using intracorporeal techniques, at the time of this writing, the
more advanced level II thrombi are performed
laparoscopic-assisted; the vena-caval exploration performed through a mini-incision. Patients with venous
involvement are generally approached using the
transperitoneal route. The use of intraoperative ultra-
sonography using a flexible, steerable laparoscopic
probe is useful in accurately mapping the extent of
tumor thrombus. Occasionally, milking the thrombus is
necessary to position the stapler distal to the tumor
thrombus in level I and very early level II cases.

References

1. Lee, D.I., Clayman, R.V.: Standard transperitoneal and laparoscopic
   nephrectomy for clinical T1-T3a, N0 and M0 Tumors. In: Laparoscopic Urologic Oncology. Edited by J.A. Cadeddu. Totowa, NJ:
   Humana Press
2. Chan, D.Y., Su, L.M., Kavoussi, L.R.: Rapid ligation of renal hilum
   during transperitoneal laparoscopic nephrectomy. Urology **57:** 360,
   2001
3. Rapp, D.E., Orvieto, M.A., Gerber, G.S., et al.: En bloc stapling of
   renal hilum during laparoscopic nephrectomy and nephroureterectomy. Urology **64:** 655, 2004

Chapter 6
Renal Cysts

What Are Your Tips on Laparoscopic Management of Suspicious Renal Cysts?

Drs. Bellman and Shpall

Our approach to renal cysts has evolved with the advent of laparoscopic partial nephrectomies. More and more often, we either excise the cyst if we are worried about it, or if not, we just leave it alone. This works well as long as the cysts are not endophytic and are amenable to resection; fortunately, most cysts are peripheral and are easily excised. For Bosniak 3 cysts, we usually recommend excision. For Bosniak 2 cysts, we will talk to the patient about the low incidence of malignancy, and help them decide between observation and excision, basing our decision on their age, co-morbidities, and preference. Typically, when a confident diagnosis of Bosniak 2 cyst can be made on CT, surgical intervention is not warranted.

What Precautions Do You Take in Avoiding Spillage Whenever You Are Laparoscopically Aspirating the Cysts?

Since we have been more aggressive in treating suspicious cysts with partial nephrectomy, we are rarely faced with aspirating anything other than Bosniak 1 cysts. Technically, it is nice if you have a laparoscopic ultrasound, and the approach is easier if the cyst is exophytic. If we were going to unroof the cyst, we would use a needle to aspirate flid for cytology, and then carefully deroof the cyst. We would then inspect the base, and fulgurate with the argon beam. If you aspirate straw- or clear-colored flid, it usually is a good indication that you are dealing with a benign entity. However, there have been two cases where the cysts were essentially normal in appearance, except for a small focus of tumor found at the base. In both of these cases, the cytology of the aspirated flid was negative. Therefore, whenever you are going to use this approach, it is important to be very fastidious in one's inspection to rule out the presence of a cystic carcinoma. We have no experience with cryoablation or radiofrequency ablation in the management of these lesions.

What Do You Do If the Cyst Is More Posterior?

We have struggled with posterior cysts, yet managed to get them done transperitoneally by thoroughly mobilizing the kidney. We certainly think a retroperitoneal approach is something to think about for a posterior cyst. We don't do much retroperitoneal surgery, but there have been times when we had wished we had chosen this approach.

Chapter 7
Partial Nephrectomy

What Are the Ways in Which You Minimize *Warm Ischemia Time?*

Dr. Gill

The most important thing is to have the requisite experience and confidence in time-sensitive and precise intracorporeal suturing. The second most important thing is to make sure everything is lined up before you clamp the renal hilum. Therefore, I go through a mental check list of seven things before I clamp the hilum:

1. The hilum has been prepared and the tumor ultrasonographically evaluated and circumferentially scored with a J-hook.
2. My pelvicaliyceal sutures (2-0 Vicryl® on CT-1 needle) and renal parenchymal sutures (0-Vicryl on CTX needle) are ready and greased.
3. The ureteral catheter is connected with syringe filled with dilute indigo carmine.
4. Intravenous mannitol has been administered five minutes prior.
5. Two bolsters are ready. Although initially in our experience, I used to preload the bolster and the sutures into the abdominal cavity, we no longer feel this is necessary. It takes barely 1 to 2 seconds to get the suture in through the port and the fewer sutures within the abdomen at any given time, the less the chances of confusion.
6. The Floseal® is ready.
7. I have a good mental picture of the angles that are required for excision of the tumor and sutured reconstruction. If the available port sites do not provide a good enough angle for either excision along the depths of the tumor or subsequent suturing, additional ports are placed as necessary. In this manner, once the hilum is clamped, no time is wasted on non-essential things. We typically cross-clamp the entire hilum *en bloc with a Satinsky clamp*. Once suturing is initiated, it is done deliberately, slowly, and precisely (Figure 7.1).

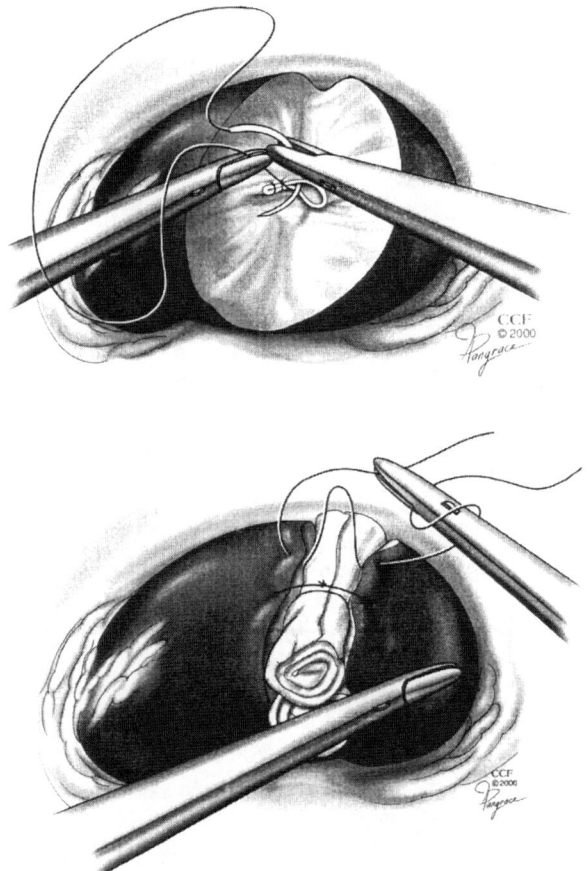

Fig. 7.1 Technique of partial nephrectomy.

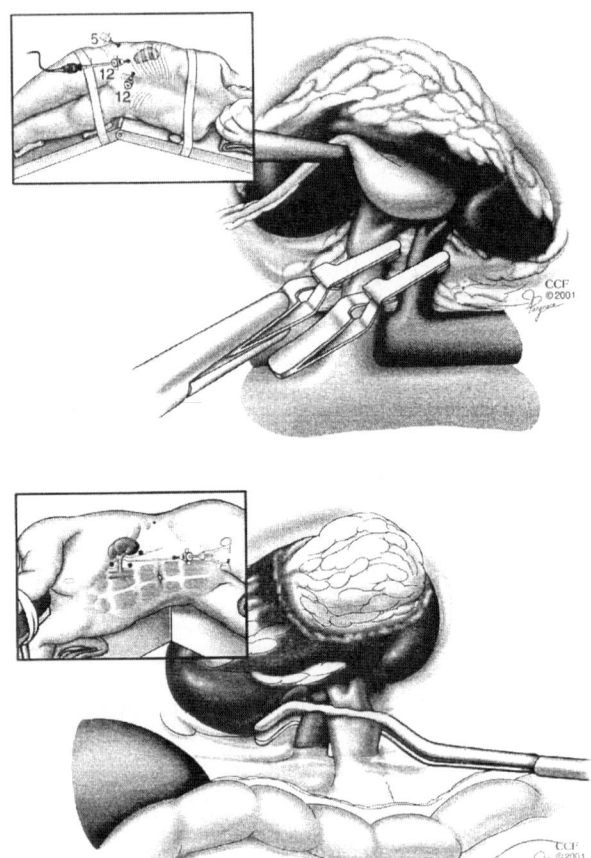

Fig. 7.1 *Continued*

What Is Your Technique of Hemostasis during Laparoscopic Partial Nephrectomy?

Dr. Gill

Our technique of hemostasis, validated in over 550 personal cases of laparoscopic partial nephrectomy, is straightforward and simple: just duplicate open surgical techniques and principles! They work well during open surgery and they work well during laparoscopy. As such, the hilum is clamped; the tumor is excised with cold endoshears in a controlled and bloodless operative field. Parenchymal hemostasis and pelvicaliyceal repair are achieved with intracorporeal suturing and renal parenchymal reconstruction is performed over a bolster with the adjunctive use of the biologic hemostatic agent Floseal®. Using this approach, our current incidence of hemorrhage and urine leak are less than 3% and 1%, respectively. And this includes advanced laparoscopic partial nephrectomies for central tumors, hilar tumors, completely intrarenal tumors, and tumors in a solitary kidney. We believe that other non-sutured techniques are unlikely to be successful as the sole hemostatic maneuver in the setting of a substantive laparoscopic partial nephrectomy.

Dr. Wolf

Over the years we have changed our approach for hemostasis during laparoscopic partial nephrectomy. We originally described a "sutureless" approach, and one that involved primarily hand assistance. We devised a hemostatic "sandwich" of fibrin glue (Tisseel®, Baxter, Deerfield, IL) and gelatin sponge (Gelfoam®, Pharmacia and Upjohn, Kalamazoo, MI) to plug defects in the kidney, staunch bleeding, and seal the collecting system. To make the hemostatic sandwich, first infiltrate a large piece of gelatin sponge with the fibrinogen component of fibrin glue, using the syringe and needle that come in the fibrin glue kit. Once the sponge is soaked with fibrinogen, place it within the abdomen wrapped up in a segment of sterile glove to prevent activation by tissue factors. Once the partial nephrectomy is done, press the fibrinogen-soaked gelatin sponge into the defect and then squirt thrombin into it using a laparoscopic cholecystostomy needle, which sets up the fibrin glue (Figure 7.2). Fibrin glue has always been a powerful hemostatic agent, but the problem is that it takes 30 seconds or so to polymerize.

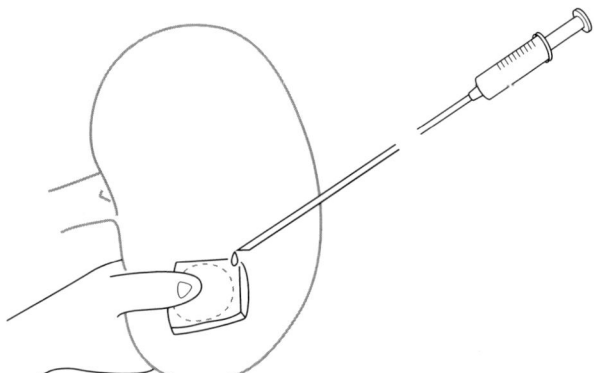

Fig. 7.2 "Hemostatic sandwich" for partial nephrectomy.

In an actively bleeding wound, fibrin glue alone gets washed away before it can do anything. With the fibrin glue/gelatin sponge composite, however, the sponge holds the fibrin glue in place while it is setting up. This fibrin glue/gelatin sponge composite can be effective in an actively bleeding wound where fibrin glue alone would be ineffective. A limitation of this hemostatic sandwich is that it is most effective with hand-assisted procedures. If it is used in standard laparoscopy, the fibrinogen-soaked sponge needs to be rolled up to fit through a port and then it sticks together and cannot be unrolled well. An alternative that can be used with standard laparoscopy is a composite of thrombin and gelatin granules (Floseal®, Baxter, Deerfield, IL). This slurry also stays in place while coagulation sets up—although the only fibrinogen in the compound is autologous (blood from the hemorrhaging) and this composite is probably not as hemostatic as the fibrin glue/gelatin sponge one.

After our first 75 procedures we examined our results and realized that this technique was inadequate in many cases.[1] Among 58 of the 75 patients in whom the resection did not enter the collecting system and/or renal sinus, the rate of postoperative hemorrhage and/or urinary leak was only 3.4%, but among the 17 patient with such entry the rate was 41%. We decided at that point to start using a sutured bolster technique for hemostasis, adapted from the technique of Dr. Gill. The results were much better. Among the next 25 patients, we used a sutured bolster whenever there was collecting system and/or renal sinus entry (18 patients), and thrombin/gelatin granules if there was not such entry (7 patients): the hemorrhage/leak rates were 11% and 0%, respectively. We concluded (and this is in perfect agreement with our experimental studies) that for resections that are superficial to the collecting system and/or renal sinus, fibrin glue products are adequate for hemostasis, but for deeper resections a sutured bolster is recommended.

Our modifications of Dr. Gill's technique are minor, but we feel that they are quite helpful. We use the same rolled bolster made of Surgicel Nu-Knit® (Johnson & Johnson, New Brunswick, NJ). We use the same 0-polyglycolic sutures, albeit with CT-1 needles (smaller than CT needles used by Dr. Gill), and the same Hem-o-lock® clips (Weck, Raleigh, NC) to secure the bolster. The modification is that we pre-load everything. The rolled bolster is pre-loaded with a pair of 2-inch lengths of 0-polyglycolic sutures on CT-1 needles, and two or three additional 6-inch lengths of 0-polyglycolic sutures on CT-1 needles are preloaded with a Hem-o-lock clip tied onto the free end. All of these are placed into the abdomen and are ready to go when we start resecting. These pre-loads save a bit of ischemia time. Finally, we are less aggressive with closing the base of the resection site (with a running 2-0 polyglycolic acid suture on an SH needle). We do not take very deep bites at all, and perform this step only when there is wide entry of the renal sinus. Omitting this suture shortens ischemia time by 5 to 10 minutes and may reduce the risk of arteriovenous fistula.

What Is Your Experience in the Use of Tissuelink® during Laparoscopic Partial Nephrectomy?

Dr. Thomas

Our initial experience with TissueLink® has been published in the *Journal of Urology*.[2] We use it in selected cases, especially lesions that are peripheral and not too deep. These are the sort of cases where one would clamp the vessels and perform partial nephrectomy, but where I've truly found it useful is in high-risk patients with hypertension, diabetes, or a marginally functioning kidney where I don't want to clamp the vessels. In those patients, if we can avoid hilar clamping, they tend to do better in the long run.

Now, there are two types of TissueLink devices. One has a small ball, which was initially available and now there is a cutting electrode, rather like a hook. The principle with both devices is the same. With the TissueLink hook, one can get to the needed plane much easier. You can also combine its use with a regular laparoscopic scissors. With the scissors, you make an incision and coagulate with the TissueLink. However, it is a slower process. Maybe it is slower because you are a little more relaxed, because we can take our time since the renal vessels are not clamped. The sense of urgency is not there. The technology is also slower. But overall it works well. Though it is not bloodless, the beauty is that in case you have not coagulated while using the TissueLink, you can still use electrocautery to get hemostasis. It does not affect your frozen section results, even though there is a certain amount of charring. If the temperature exceeds 100°, the device won't work. So you have good margins and specimens and any criticism of not being able to get a frozen section biopsy is not true.

What Are the Optimal Angles of Port Placement to Facilitate Suturing in Renal Surgery?

Dr. Rassweiler

I must admit that we are somewhat fixed with the retroperitoneal laparoscopic approach using the Petit's triangle. The ideal angle for suturing the upper ureter, such as for pyeloplasty, must be greater than 25 degrees and it works well.[3] However, for partial nephrectomy, the ideal angle would depend on the location of the tumor. For a tumor that is on the lower pole and exophytic posteriorly, suturing is usually straightforward and we employ the retroperitoneal approach. If it is at the upper pole posteriorly, that would be an indication for a transperitoneal approach. I must admit that we are less aggressive with the decision to perform partial nephrectomy for renal tumors in comparison to the Cleveland group; so I do more radical nephrectomies than partial. For us, still, the maximum (tumor size) for partial nephrectomy is 4 cm.

Do You Place A Tourniquet around the Renal Artery?

Dr. Laguna

We have been using the laparoscopic version of the Rummel tourniquets for controlling the renal artery during the partial nephrectomy. We learned this from our Spanish friends Drs. J. Salvador and A. Rosales from Fundacion Puigvert.[4] Essentially, it consists of passing a double loop created by means of a vessel loop or a small piece of a 16 F catheter around the renal artery. Once the tourniquet is in place, a clip placed in the distal end of the catheter will stabilize and maintain the compression. After suturing the parenchyma, cutting one of the loops will free the tourniquet (Figure 7.3).

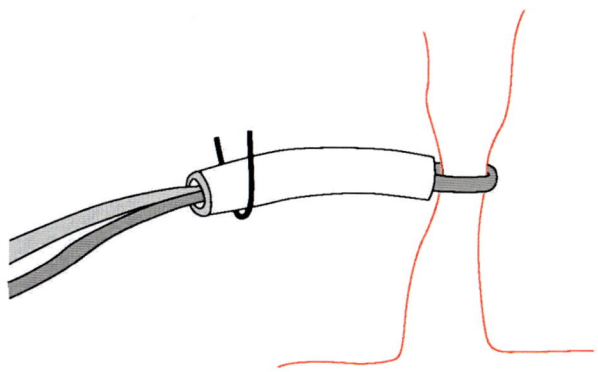

Fig. 7.3 Rummel tourniquet.

Do You Use Lapra Ty® Clips for Partial Nephrectomy?

Dr. Shalhav

The Lapra Ty® (Ethicon Endosurgery, Cincinnati, OH) is extremely useful when performing a partial nephrectomy. It is very useful to close the collecting system as well as over-sew the resection bed. In addition, the use of Lapra Ty® clips on the bolster sutures used to compress the renal parenchyma during a partial nephrectomy has revolutionized our management of laparoscopic and open partial nephrectomies. Essentially, with a Lapra Ty® clip on one end, the renal parenchyma can be easily compressed along a 180-degree plane in line with the suture (Figure 7.4). This prevents any cheese-slicing effect that can occur if the sutures are pulled at an acute angle for tying. In addition, if any of the bolster sutures is found to have too much slack, further tension can be obtained by gently pulling a loose end and placing an additional Lapra Ty® clip below the first one to further cinch down on the tissue.

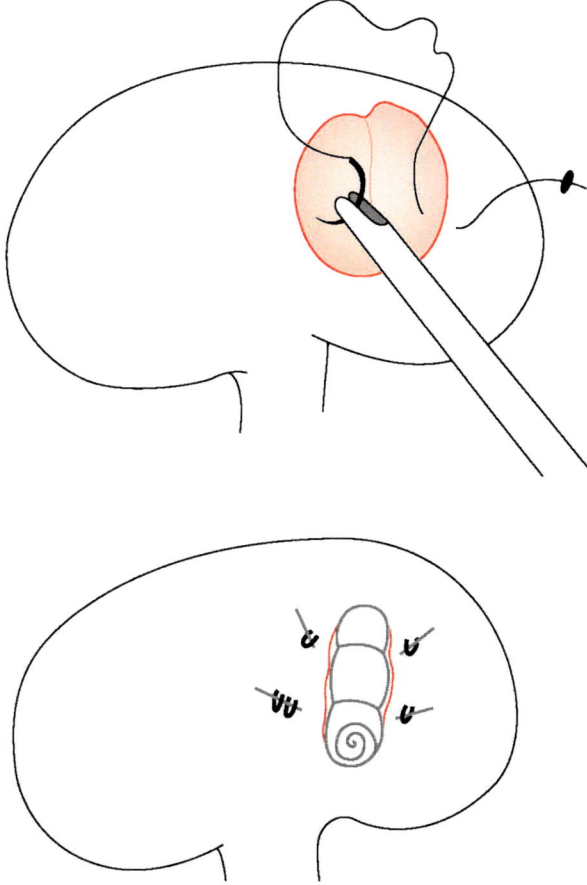

Fig. 7.4 Use of the Lapra Ty® clip for partial nephrectomy.

References

1. Johnston, W.K., 3rd, Montgomery, J.S., Seifman, B.D., et al.: Fibrin glue v. sutured bolster: lessons learned during 100 laparoscopic partial nephrectomies. J Urol **174:** 47, 2005

2. Urena, R., Mendez, F., Woods, M., et al.: Laparoscopic partial nephrectomy of solid renal masses without hilar clamping using a monopolar radio frequency device. J Urol **171:** 1054, 2004

3. Frede, T., Stock, C., Renner, C., et al.: Geometry of laparoscopic suturing and knotting techniques. J Endourol **13:** 191, 1999

4. Rosales, A., Salvador, J., De Graeve, N., et al.: Clamping of the renal artery in laparoscopic partial nephrectomy: An old device for a new technique. Eur Urol **47:** 98, 2005

Chapter 8
Radiofrequency and Cryoablation of Renal Tumors

What Are the Principles of Radiofrequency Ablation (RFA) of Renal Tumors?

Dr. Cadeddu

Patient selection is most important for RFA. Watch for surrounding landmarks. I have significant concerns for tumors that abut the collecting system, particularly tumors that abut the ureteropelvic junction.

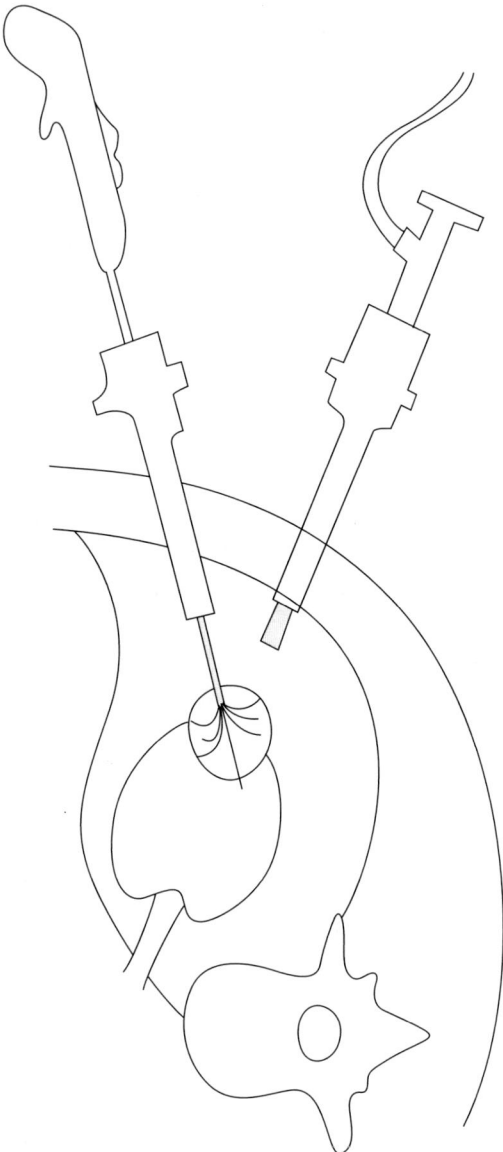

Fig. 8.1 Laparoscopic radiofrequency ablation.

Radiofrequency ablation causes ischemia of tissues and as such can result in ischemic stenosis or strictures of the collecting system. We have lost two kidneys due to such a complication. The other thing is, similar to cryoablation, you must protect the adjacent organs. If bowel is present, particularly within 5 mm or less from the lesion, I would not advise performing any ablation, without some way of protecting the bowel, either laparoscopically, or as some people have reported, by hydrodissection and instillation of saline. Ablation of adjacent liver or spleen is, in my opinion, okay because that just results in a region of ischemia of the liver or spleen which should recover without difficulty. Also, we select tumors that are less than 4 cm, though others have reported larger tumors. The physics of radiofrequency ablation would suggest that for larger than 4-cm tumors it would require multiple ablations. Also I have concerns that the biological activity of tumors is more aggressive when they are more than 4 cm, and since this a technology that has not proven long-term efficacy, I am hesitant about treating those tumors.

There is significant difference between the natural history of radiofrequency-ablated lesions versus those treated with cryoablation. In cryoablation, where the nature of creating a freeze-and-thaw cycle results in cellular lysis, the cell membranes actually rupture, and this results in spillage of cellular contents. The result is that you get infiltration of neutrophils and macrophages and reabsorption of those proteins and the mass such that within a few years the majority of the cryo-ablated lesions shrink significantly or disappear. Radiofrequency is distinctly different. The behavior of radiofrequency is similar to what one sees in the prostate: by heating tissues, it results in denaturing of proteins; cross-linking of proteins; and, in essence, solidification of the region of ablation. I use the analogy of a hard boiled egg. The result is, instead of a lysed tumor, you have a truly solid-ified tumor. The immune system, when it reacts to this no longer viable tissue, cannot infiltrate neutrophils and macrophages into the tissue, since it is cross-linked and solidified. What it does, in lay terms, is that it walls it off. Histologically there is a foreign-body reaction and you get a granuloma. You see microscopically, giant cells and literally a fibrotic ring around the tumor. So, on imaging, in cryotherapy one wants to see not only no enhancement but also shrinkage of the tumor. In RFA, one should also not see enhancement but one does not see significant shrinkage. One thing we tend to see though on long-term CT scanning and MRI scanning is the ring of fibrosis around the ablated tumor. So we have a difference in the natural history of the tumor and we have published this.[1]

How Do You Decide among RFA, Cryoablation, and Laparoscopic Partial Nephrectomy?

Dr. Cadeddu

I try not to make a decision. I try to let the patient make an informed and educated decision. I certainly believe that ablation technologies have not been demonstrated to have long-term efficacy. I do not deny that during discus-sion with the patient. So when the patient is able to make a decision intelligently, I will explain to them RF and cryoablation. Now, at our center we do radiofrequency ablation; we don't do cryoablation. But the technologies, in my mind, are the same. So with radiofrequency ablation, every person that is a candidate for radiofrequency ablation, based on the criteria I already mentioned, is also a candidate for laparoscopic partial nephrectomy. They will undergo an extensive informed-consent process that explains that radiofrequency ablation in the short term has very good efficacy, but in the long term, i.e., more than three years, we do know the natural history of these lesions. So if the patient wants definitive treatment, certainly laparoscopic partial nephrectomy is recommended. The elderly patient or a patient with significant co-morbidities or the patient with prior surgeries will obviously find radiofrequency ablation more appealing and often will choose that as an alternative. The age of the patient certainly is a big factor in deciding in favor of RF; for example, an octogenarian, may not want watchful waiting because of his fear of cancer. However I have treated people in their 40s, 50s, and 60s specifically if they have significant co-morbidities. We also see people with cardiac disease and diabetes and a solitary kidney and they may have chosen radiofrequency ablation, but age is certainly a driving factor.

What Are the Technical Nuances of Laparoscopic Renal Cryoablation?

Dr. Gill

The location of the tumor determines the laparoscopic approach: posterior and lateral tumors are approached retroperitoneally, while anterior tumors are approached transperitoneally. Following ultrasonographic localization, the dimensions of the tumor are measured, including tumor depth (Figure 8.2). The tumor depth is then marked on the cryoprobe with sterile ink, thereby giving a visual idea as to how deep the probe has to be inserted into the tumor, so as to have the probe tip at or just beyond the inner margin of the tumor. Under sonographic control, the cryoprobe is inserted in a perpendicular manner to the center of the tumor and precisely advanced with a gradual twisting manner to the exact desired depth. Probe overshoot must not occur. To

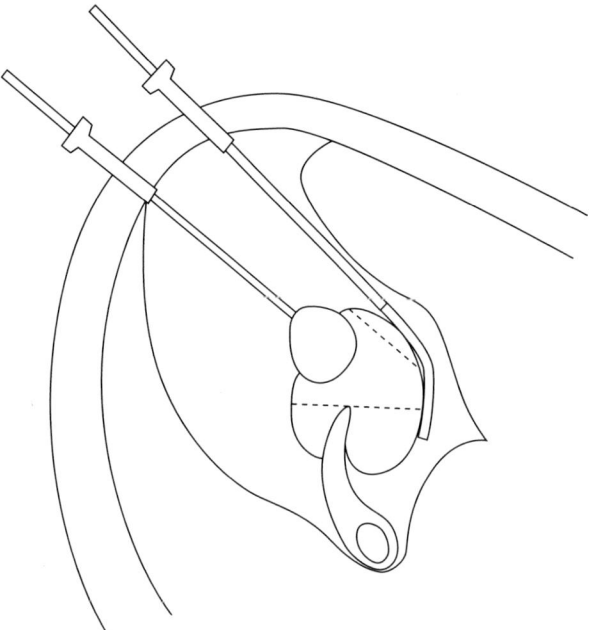

Fig. 8.2 Laparoscopic renal cryoablation.

facilitate the initial puncture of the tumor surface, the intended puncture sire of the tumor site can be breached by a J-hook electrocautery application, thereby making probe insertion easier. The evolving cryolesion is then monitored by the dual control of laparoscopic visualization, which monitors the extra-renal aspect of the ice ball, and ultrasonographic guidance, which monitors the intra-renal part of the ice ball. To achieve this, the ultrasound probe must be placed in contact with the opposite surface of the kidney. We typically use a 4.8-mm cryoprobe and reserve cryoablation for tumors that are no larger than 3 cm in size. For larger tumors, two or more probes may be necessary. The ice ball is usually extended one cm beyond the laparoscopically and ultrasonographically visible extent of the tumor circumferentially. A double freeze–thaw cycle is performed. Extreme care is taken to ensure that neither the cryolesion nor the active cryoprobe comes in contact with any adjacent structure or viscera at any time during the procedure. Contact of the ice ball with the ureter, bowel, or other abdominal viscera will almost certainly produce a transmural cryoinjury, resulting in severe sequela such as ureteral stricture, bowel fistula, bowel obstruction, etc. Manipulating the cryoprobe while it is firmly engaged within the ice ball has the potential to set up parenchymal fracture lines, which may result in postoperative hemorrhage. Upon completion of cryoablation, the ice ball must be allowed to thaw completely. Only when the cryoprobe is fully released as confirmed by gentle twisting movement of the cryoprobe, should the cryoprobe be disengaged. Hemostasis of the probe track in the kidney parenchyma can be obtained by using Floseal® and/or argon beam coagulation. When using argon beam coagulation, one should be cognizant that argon embolus can potentially occur if the ABC beam is directly focused on an open intra-parenchymal blood vessel.

What Are Your Three Tips for Renal Cryotherapy?

Dr. Nakada

The first one is you always want to have good case selection, and that in itself is a book chapter. What we generally prefer right now is the laparoscopic approach; with an anterior or a lateral tumor we will go transperitoneal, and if it is otherwise we will go retroperitoneal. I believe most of these cases will eventually be percutaneous. One tip is that I tend to use a larger probe and create a single ice ball. You are going to have your best freeze in the central region, and at the margins you will have possibly less effective cell death. So I prefer the large ice ball rather than the multiple small ice balls created by the needle system, because then I believe that you are putting yourself at risk for multiple potential margins. So when possible, use a larger probe and thus a larger ice ball, as I think that is a more effective approach.

Another tip: the collecting system is relatively resistant to cryoinjury. So unlike radiofrequency ablation, you do not have to be quite as worried about injuring the collecting system. Obviously, you are under ultrasound guidance and some folks have reported using a warm irrigant to protect the collecting system, but in fact you may be compromising your margins. I would err on the side of getting a good margin. That might not be quite the case with the renal hilum.

The third tip for cryo is, if you can, you should work with an ultrasonographer when you do it laparoscopically, because really how accurate you are with the procedure is going to be directly related to the quality of your imaging. So we have one ultrasonographer who works with us on all of our laparoscopic cryo cases.

Dr. Kaouk

Do not hesitate to insert more than one cryoprobe if the renal tumor is larger than 3 cm.

The tip of the cryoprobe should be at the inner margin of the tumor. Besides ultrasound confirmation of the cryoprobe position, the resistance felt while advancing the cryoprobe onto the inner tumor capsule may be a helpful clue that the tip of the cryoprobe is at the inner margin of the tumor. All probes should be inserted prior to initiation of freezing. If the renal tumor is central and the ice ball did include part of the renal collecting system, then a JP drain should be placed for a short period (removed when drainage is <50 cc)

Give enough time for the ice ball to thaw completely prior to confirmation of hemostasis. If bleeding continues at the site of cryoprobe puncture after application of argon coagulation and Floseal®, then check other sites of bleeding such as hilar area and dissected Gerota's fat.

Apply a Surgicel® and constant pressure till the hemostasis is secured.

Reference

1. Matsumoto, E.D., Watumull, L., Johnson, D.B., et al.: The radiographic evolution of radio frequency ablated renal tumors. J Urol **172:** 45, 2004

Chapter 9
Pyeloplasty

What Are Some Tips for Laparoscopic Pyeloplasty?

Dr. Eden

As far as pyeloplasty is concerned, the best advice is to do it extraperitoneally. It is much more direct and it brings you, whether you are doing a left- or a right-sided case, really right up to the ureteropelvic junction (UPJ), since the collecting system is the most lateral structure. Compared to the transperitoneal approach, dissection of the crossing vessels is easier, but the anastomosis is a bit more difficult because you are sewing around the vessels. The rest of the operation is much easier.

I guess one of the things that I have seen people struggle most with, which takes me very little time, is the pelvic reduction and the spatulation of the ureter. What I do if I want to reduce the pelvis is to excise the pelvis with the UPJ not dismembered, so that the pelvis is completely stabilized (Figure 9.1). Incise where you want to make the most proximal incision, excise a disc of renal pelvis, and then remove it. You then dismember the UPJ, grasp the ureter on the most lateral aspect, and pull it toward you and down. It is very important to hold the ureter in a straight line so that you are then looking down the mouth of the ureter. Next, insert one blade of the scissors into the open ureter, close the blades and you have spatulated the ureter over 1 cm. It is extremely quick and much faster than most of the techniques I have seen others use.

As far as anastomosis is concerned, you should always start with the heel (Figure 9.2). You should place three

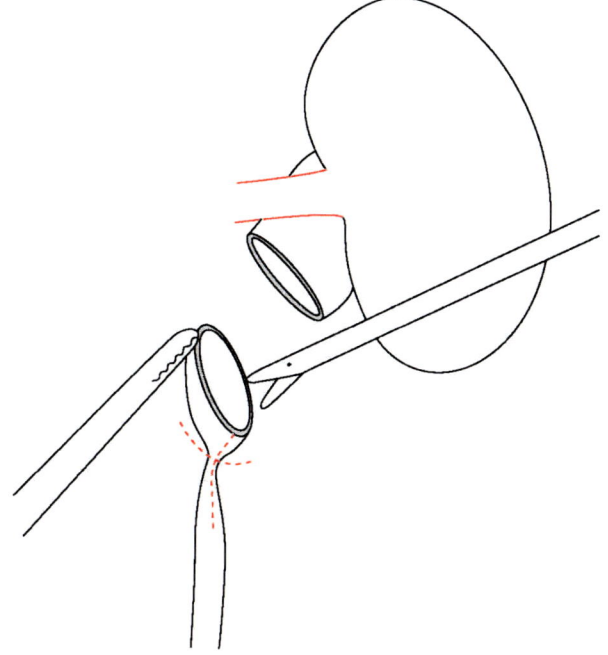

Fig. 9.1 Spatulation of ureter.

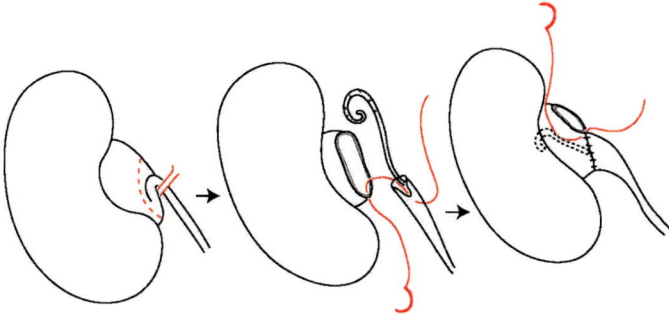

Fig. 9.2 Dismembered pyeloplasty.

sutures at the heel before doing anything else, because if you are going to have a urine leak from the pyeloplasty this is where it is going to be. It is best to put those sutures in right at the beginning when you have the best view of the tissue edges. You need to suture with 3 mm bites of tissue, 3 mm apart. I think they need to be interrupted because the ureter has a longitudinal blood supply, which is relatively tenuous. If you use a continuous suture material, at least in theory, you have more risk of ischemia. I always suture the uretero-pelvic anastomosis interrupted and then use a running suture to close the pelvis if I have reduced it. Running sutures require the use of a monofilament, such as Monocryl®. If you use a braided suture you may find that when you pull up at the end of the suturing, the tension of the suture does not equalize across its length. In other words, you won't have all the tissue opposed. Braided sutures also create more tissue trauma through drag and so are not as well-suited as monofilament sotores when used in a continuous fashion.

Dr. Kumar

To retract the ureter during pyeloplasty, one may need to grasp it gently with a grasper. But this often "uses up" a port. One way of retracting the ureter is to use a suture on Keith needle passed through the abdominal wall under endoscopic vision hooking below the ureter and then brought out to the skin. The suture may then be placed on tension as necessary to elevate the ureter (Figure 9.3).

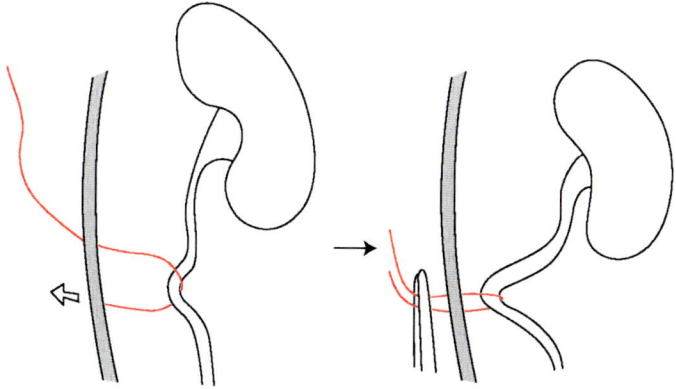

Fig. 9.3 A technique for retraction of the ureter.

What Are Your Views on Fengerplasty?

Dr. Kumar

While dismembered pyeloplasty is the standard procedure for ureteropelvic junction obstruction, a non-dismembered pyeloplasty using the Heineke–Mickulicz principle may be employed in select patients (Figure 9.4). In this procedure, the ureteropelvic junction is opened vertically and sutured in a transverse direction using three or four interrupted sutures to create a wider opening. The advantage is that it is much easier to perform. However, this must be used only when there are no crossing lower pole vessels or if such vessels are present, the reconstructed UPJ must be positioned well below the level of the vessels by mobilization of the redundant pelvis.

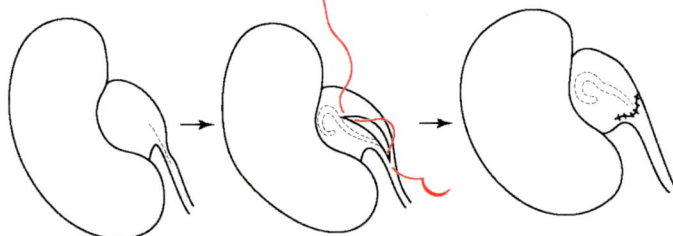

Fig. 9.4 Fengerplasty.

Do You Place A Ureteral Stent Prior to Pyeloplasty?

Dr. Kumar

There are several suggestions for stent/ureteral catheter placement prior to performing laparoscopic pyeloplasty. It is generally agreed that the presence of a stent at the time of the ureteral dissection makes it easier to identify the ureter. However, the presence of a stent for prolonged period of days or weeks prior to the pyeloplasty can result in inflammation and edema of the ureter, making suturing difficult. We therefore routinely recommend removal of any previously placed ureteral stent several days before the surgery, unless there are overriding reasons not to do so.

Prior to the pyeloplasty, I perform a flexible cystoscopy in the supine position and place a guidewire under fluoroscopic guidance. An open-ended ureteric catheter is then passed over the guidewire after removal of the cystoscope, a retrograde ureterogram performed, and the catheter is positioned with its tip a few centimeters below the UPJ. It is helpful to have a distended renal pelvis for easier dissection and for that reason I do not pass the catheter all the way into the pelvis. A urethral Foley catheter is placed, and the ureteric catheter is secured to the foley catheter. The patient is then repositioned for the laparoscopic pyeloplasty in a 60-degree lateral position. The ureteric catheter is included in the sterile preparation of the abdomen and kept in the field for access during surgery.

During dissection of the retroperitoneum, the ureteric catheter may be manipulated to help identify the ureter. Absence of a stent across the UPJ also makes it easier to divide the UPJ for pyeloplasty. Once one is ready to have the stent placed across the repair, a guidewire, passed through the ureteral catheter in a retrograde fashion, is brought out through one of the ports, the ureteral catheter is removed, and the ureteral stent is then passed antegradely and positioned in the pelvis prior to completion of the anastomosis.

Dr. de la Rosette

We initially were stenting all the patients during the surgery, either retrograde or using laparoscopic guidance, but that caused a lot of difficulties and problems. So we decided to insert a stent on the day prior to surgery. First of all, you are not pressed for time; and secondly, by having a very nice retrograde study, any other abnormalities are detected. So you can avoid problems during the surgery. So pre-stenting with a double-J stent facilitates the surgery in all respects.

Drs. Bellman and Shpall

We always place the ureteral stent beforehand. We have looked at different techniques, and certainly one has to be careful when one does a dismembered pyeloplasty, not to cut the stent (it has happened a few times)! When we *have* inadvertently cut the stent, we have removed both pieces of the damaged stent, maneuvered a guidewire into the bladder, and passed a new stent, ensuring that the distal coil is within the bladder. We then continue with the remainder of the pyeloplasty. The stent does sometimes get in the way of our suturing, but usually we are able to work around it. We use a slightly longer, 6 French stent.

We leave the stent in two to three weeks. We used to use fibrin glue over the anastomosis, but have recently stopped this practice. We always leave a flank drain. We remove the Foley catheter after one day; if output increases from the flank drain, we will replace the Foley.

What Are Your Three Tips for Laparoscopic Pyeloplasty?

Dr. Gill

1. It does not really matter whether one places a double-J stent in the ureter retrogradely preoperatively using cystoscopy, or intraoperatively in an antegrade manner by laparoscopic techniques. We have employed both approaches and both work equally well.

2. In our experience, the optimum stent is a 4.7 French 26-cm stent. A stent of larger diameter occupies the ureteral lumen substantially, making it difficult to place ureteral stitches. The 4.7 French stent allows the needle to be placed efficiently alongside the stent when taking ureteral bites. A 26-cm stent typically works in all patients to have both curls in the appropriate places in the bladder and renal pelvis. *Also, one can instill 200 cc of saline with indigo carmine into the bladder. As soon as the antegradely inserted double-J stent enters the bladder, reflux up the stent is noted and leakage of blue dye from the stent confirms that the distal coil is in the bladder.*

3. In discussions with my pediatric urology colleagues, we do not believe that it is important to excise the stenotic ureteropelvic junction area. The most important elements are wide spatulation of the ureter and the pelvis and precise mucosa-to-mucosa anastomosis in a tension-free manner. As such, the ureteropelvic junction is excised only if adequate ureteral redundant length is available.

Dr. Thomas

1. We place an open-ended ureteral catheter just prior to the procedure and place it just distal to the UPJ. The reason for doing this is that sometimes patients are sent to us with a stent. When the stent is in place, you always find that the stent is in the way of our incision of the UPJ. Also, it drains the renal pelvis, so you don't have a dilated renal pelvis. I would like the renal pelvis to be distended. I remove the stent and place a

ureteral catheter up to the UPJ. This distends the obstructed renal pelvis without draining it (because of the UPJO) and I can get to the UPJ much quicker after reflecting the colon. We recommend this technique in pediatrics, as well as in older patients. The second advantage to having the open-ended catheter up to the UPJ is that, intraoperatively, I am able to manipulate a super-stiff guidewire to place a stent in a retrograde manner. It works easily without losing pneumoperitoneum as with going antegrade through a trocar.

2. Trick number two is to place our working port subxiphoid. I've seen other people do it differently, placing it either in the right- or left-lower quadrant, but we find that this is not user-friendly. The subxiphoid location is a straight shot to the UPJ, so we can deliver the suture, remove the needle, perform suction, or perform a flexible nephroscopy/ureteroscopy if there are associated stones.

3. The third modification that we recommend is, in cases of UPJO secondary to crossing vessels, one needs to perform a very adequate pelviolysis. This is why keeping the pelvis distended (Trick 1) helps with the dissection just as one would with a hydrocele sac. Besides, when it is distended, I know exactly how much I need to reduce the renal pelvis; how much of it needs to be dissected over, under, and around the crossing vessels; and that does help me tremendously in moving the UPJ distally and away from the main renal vessels or any crossing vessels. This third point, again, is to recommend an adequate renal pelvic and UPJ lysis.

Do You Prefer Continued Versus Interrupted Sutures for Laparoscopic Pyeloplasty?

Dr. Gill

I prefer two continuous sutures. A 4-0 suture on an RB-1 needle is employed. The anastomosis is always performed from the apex of the ureteral spatulation toward the pelvis with the initial stitch being placed at the apex. I initially run the posterior wall of the anastomosis and then use a second stitch to run the anterior wall of the anastomosis. At the conclusion of the anastomosis, 10 mg of *Lasix and an ampoule of indigo carmine* are administered intravenously to assess the water tightness of the anastomosis.

Do You Use the Lapra Ty® Clip for Pyeloplasties?

Dr. Shalhav

Yes, I typically run two separate sutures along the anterior and posterior lines of the anastomosis. After spatulating the ureter along its lateral aspect, I begin by suturing the posterior anastomosis first followed by the anterior anastomosis. Suture lines are run from a lateral to medial direction. At the starting point laterally, which is the narrowest point, I intracorporeally tie these sutures ensuring the knot is on the outside. However, at

the end of the suture line on the medial aspect, I use the
Lapra Ty® clip to anchor each suture on the renal
pelvis. This concept is not new, as Ralph Clayman previously published the use of the Lapra Ty® clip during a
pyeloplasty as early as 1995. However, in his series, a
Lapra Ty® clip was used on each end of the suture
line, which I don't like to do. Although the Lapra Ty® clip
is biodegradable, I prefer not to use it on the lateral
aspect, where I feel the anastomosis is most delicate.
During to the six- to eight-week period for theoretical
absorption of these clips, inflammation may develop
at the suture line along with possible scarring. Therefore,
I only use these clips along the medial aspect of each
anastomosis.

How Do You Handle Crossing Vessels?

Dr. Gill

A crossing renal vein can be sacrificed if it is a non-dominant vein of the kidney. A crossing renal artery must
always be preserved. The ureter and UPJ area are completely dissected free from the crossing vessel both
cephalad and caudal to the vessel. The UPJ area is then
transected in an angled manner and the pyeloplasty
anastomosis is completed. It is important to ensure that
at the conclusion of the operation, the crossing vessel
does not directly lie across the reconstructed UPJ. If it
does, the vessel can be tacked cephalad with a stitch and
adjacent perirenal fat can be interposed between the
ureter and the crossing vessel.

In Patients with a Crossing Vessel, Do You Routinely Transpose the Vessels?

Dr. Gill

No. This decision is made on an individual basis dictated by the lie of the vessels and the ureter. In our experience, when performing a transperitoneal pyeloplasty, it is quite difficult to reconstruct the ureter posterior to the crossing vessel. As such, typically one ends up transposing the ureter anterior to the crossing vessels. Conversely, during the retroperitoneal laparoscopic pyeloplasty, it is similarly difficult to anastomose the UPJ anterior to the crossing vessels, since the retroperitoneal approach visualizes the renal artery and vessels first and the ureter next. As such, one typically ends up leaving the ureter posterior to the renal vessels. Most laparoscopic surgeons will tell you that they routinely transpose the ureter, but I believe that is more a reflection of the fact that most laparoscopists employ the transperitoneal approach for a laparoscopic pyeloplasty. We have compared outcomes in patients with and without ureteral transposition, and there is no difference.

Dr. Stoller

The etiology of the renal ureteropelvic junction obstruction is unknown. What is the contribution of crossing vessels and what is the contribution of ureteral and pelvic intrinsic muscular insufficiency? We do realize that crossing vessels have a significant impact on the success rates when you do a retrograde or antegrade endopyelotomy.

Early in my experience, we found a few cases with a very small intrarenal pelvis and a very tight band of vessels, and I felt that it would be very difficult to perform a laparoscopic pyeloplasty. I mobilized the vessels all the way from their insertion into the renal parenchyma to their insertion in the great vessels. I then used a hammock or a sling fashioned from either perirenal Gerota's fascia or omental tissue around the vessels to transpose the vessel high up in a more cephalad position to allow the UPJ to be independent of the crossing vessels. The conclusion from my early experience is that maybe we should do this more often. We've now done 15 cases without doing anything to the UPJ and had excellent long-term results. The question that arises is, At what point do you intervene to determine whether there is an intrinsic obstruction of the UPJ versus just a crossing vessel? If the UPJ looks like a nice funnel and you can see the peristalsis going down into the ureter, then translocation of the vessels without transecting the ureter may be a viable option. Hellstrom described it initially during traditional open surgery and reported good success. It is not for every patient and is dependent on intraoperative observations to decide whether the Hellstrom procedure is a viable option. I think the success of the Hellstrom procedure helps us better understand that crossing vessels may be the primary etiology for a select group of patients with UPJO.

Dr. Thomas

The need for transposition is a very controversial one and has been debated at length, because, depending on the literature, crossing vessels are encountered in anywhere from 22% to 60% of patients. Most crossing vessels can now be diagnosed preoperatively, especially with advanced diagnostic imaging techniques. The question is, Do you really need to mess with the vessels at all? How do you deal with the vessels? Some people suggest transposing the vessels like the Hellstrom technique, which I have not done because I am concerned about kinking the vessels. Should we move the pelvis in front or away from the vessels? I don't usually transpose the renal pelvis. The reason is that once I perform an adequate pelviolysis, I am able to move the UPJ away from where the "incriminating" blood vessel or band is. I have found the need for transposing the vessels just twice in the last 64 consecutive UPJs and, in my experience, 36 (55%) of these had crossing vessels. Now, all of the crossing vessels may not necessarily be significant but some *were* significant. I don't tend to move the anastomosis anteriorly because you can perform an adequate pelviolysis and move the UPJ distally away from where you thought the vessel was causing pressure. Thus, your anastomosis is way caudad to these vessels. The second reason, if you look at the dynamics of the renal pelvis, if you now transpose it over the vessels, you are not sure whether you are causing any secondary obstruction. Preoperatively, the vessel is anterior to the UPJ and compressing it, and if you transpose the UPJ anterior to the vessels, then do you have enough length without causing tension and then are you creating possible secondary obstruction? We've been following our robotic and laparoscopic experiences very closely with a combination of urograms, renal scans, ultrasounds, and CT scans, and we really haven't had a true failure. We've had one patient who had significant hydrocalicosis that went from severe to moderate improvement, but the patient is asymptomatic and I think that was the best that could be done. That is my theory on crossing vessels. This is also my reason for leaving the renal pelvis distended, as it allows me to perform an adequate pelviolysis and move the renal pelvis and UPJ caudad.

When You Do A Dismembered Pyeloplasty, Do You Transpose the Vessels or Not?

Dr. Stoller

Yes, I do. If you are going to do a dismembered pyeloplasty, you might as well just move the vessel from an anterior to a posterior location. But if you are not going to do a dismembered pyeloplasty, say, you are going to do a Y-V plasty or you're going to do a Fengerplasty, which is popular in Europe, then maybe the combination (of the repair and the Hellstrom transposition) may be worthwhile. I think that persistent pulsation of the vessels across the repair can be avoided in this fashion. There was also a report at the World Congress of Endourology in Mumbai, where they transected the crossing vein but not the artery without any other intervention. They found that it worked fine, so I think this is a concept that may be applied to laparoscopic procedures.

Any Tips for Suturing in Pyeloplasty?

Dr. Eden

It is extremely important always to use a pair of matched needle holders that you are used to. It is also important to get facile with suturing with both the left and right hands as soon as possible. For a laparoscopic left pyeloplasty, I always suture the entire anastomosis with my left hand, because the tissues lend themselves to this best. For right-sided pyeloplasty, I would suture with my right hand.

In terms of ergonomics, I certainly don't think it is always important to try to triangulate the instruments. Indeed, in extraperitoneal renal laparoscopy you can't always triangulate the instruments; they are almost parallel to each other. This really doesn't matter. You can still suture very easily for an extraperitoneal pyeloplasty and it really isn't a problem. If it is a long case, such as re-do surgery, or if you are early in your laparoscopic experience, I think it is very important to be comfortable. You need to stand up straight, with your elbows at 90 degrees. Your assistant also needs to be comfortable, either standing or seated and I think it is very important to make sure that your elbows are not at the same level. So if your assistant isn't seated, then it is important to get him to stand on a platform, just so that your elbows aren't constantly clashing.

When you're suturing during a prostatectomy, and it took me a long time to discover this, it is much more comfortable if you stand on a platform. Your shoulders, especially your deltoid muscles get much less tired and then you can truly suture with your intrinsic hand muscles instead of your upper arm muscles, allowing greater precision.

How Do You Decide between Dismembered and Non-dismembered Pyeloplasty?

Drs. Bellman and Shpall

We only perform dismembered pyeloplasties.

Is There a Case for Doing a Non-dismembered Pyeloplasty in Your Opinion?

Drs. Bellman and Shpall

I've looked at those techniques and I've considered them, but when I've been in the operating room actually doing the case, I have usually erred on the side of doing dismemberment and totally excising the segment; it makes mc feel better! I do think that there are some patients who have a short segment of obstruction that probably would do fine with a non-dismembered procedure, though I've continued to do dismembered pyeloplasties almost routinely.

Any Technical Tips about Appropriate Port Placement for the Suturing?

Drs. Bellman and Shpall

I think it is important to get good mobilization of the renal pelvis so that you have a tension-free anastomosis. Usually we use the umbilicus for the camera port but sometimes we use the lower mid-clavicular line port. For additional port placements we will use two 5-mm ports, one posterior and one anterior, which are used for suturing.

What Sort of Suture Material Do You Use?

Drs. Bellman and Shpall

We now use interrupted 4–0 Vicryl®. In the past, we had used an absorbable monofilament suture, such as PDS®; however, the inherent memory of this suture material caused curling and kinking, which unnecessarily increased the technical difficulty of the anastamosis.

When You Say You Place A Stay Suture, Where Do You Place It?

Drs. Bellman and Shpall

We spatulate the ureter and place our first suture between the apex and the renal pelvis. Once tied, we use that as our stay suture to help expose the anterior and posterior surfaces of the ureter and pelvis. We place a row of interrupted sutures on the posterior aspect, then flip the stay suture around and complete the anastamosis anteriorly.

Chapter 10
Adrenalectomy

Are there Points Specific to Laparoscopic Pheochromocytoma Surgery?

Dr. Gill

An excellent preoperative medical preparation of the patient is the key. We typically optimize the patient with calcium channel blockers, with secondary use of alpha-

1 blockers and beta blockers in select circumstances. Cardiovascular clearance is essential. Vigorous intravenous hydration, early control of the adrenal vein, and minimal handling of the tumor are essential aspects of surgery. If adequate experience with retroperitoneoscopy is not available, the transperitoneal approach should be preferred in that circumstance. At our institution, we would approach the adrenal pheochromocytoma either transperitoneally or retroperitoneally without any general preference for either approach. Another key approach to adrenal surgery is to stay outside the periadrenal fat, thereby minimizing or completely avoiding handling of the adrenal gland per se, which will uniformly lead to adrenal gland fracture with troublesome hemorrhage.

What are Some Pointers to Identify the Adrenal Vein During Laparoscopy?

Dr. Suzuki

On the left side, it is important to secure wide exposure of the adrenal gland by adequately mobilizing the spleen. This is done by dividing the peritoneal attachments of the spleen all the way to the greater curvature of the stomach. We endeavor always to mobilize the spleen in this manner, because once so mobilized, the spleen falls away from the operative field and provides excellent exposure of the upper pole of the kidney and adrenal.[1]

Initially, we do not seek the adrenal vein itself. We identify the landmarks around the upper pole of the kidney, including the diaphragm, transversus muscle, and quadratus lumborum muscle; and medial to the adrenal, the posterior surface of the pancreas is identified. Following delineation of the above structures, the adrenal vein can be identified. However, if the adrenal vein is to be identified early, we dissect close to the renal hilum, opening the Gerota's fascia. The renal vein can be then identified and then the adrenal vein along its upper border. But, unless indicated, my preference is to dissect and secure the adrenal vein last; as otherwise, it can lead to congestion of the adrenal gland.

On the right side, it is fairly easy to identify the adrenal vein. As on the left side, we initially identify and demarcate the other structures near the superior pole of the kidney including the diaphragm, transversus muscle, quadratus lumborum muscle, and medially the inferior vena cava. The vena cava is an important landmark. The short hepatic vein that drains into the vena cava is a good guide to the adrenal vein, as it lies very close to it and is almost at the same level. But similar to the left side, we prefer to dissect the adrenal vein following the dissection of the gland itself.

What are the Key Technical Maneuvers During a Laparoscopic Transperitoneal Adrenalectomy?

Dr. Gill

The single-most-important thing for me is the anatomic fact that the left main adrenal vein exits the infero-

medial edge of the left adrenal gland and courses medially and obliquely to enter the renal vein (Figure 10.1).
Typically, after reflecting the left colon, the gonadal vein
can be followed cephalad to identify the renal vein. The
gonadal vein almost always enters the renal vein somewhat laterally compared to the entry point of the left
adrenal vein. Therefore, on reaching the left renal vein
along the gonadal vein, dissection is performed medially
along the anterior surface of the renal vein to identify
the left adrenal vein. The left adrenal vein is doubly

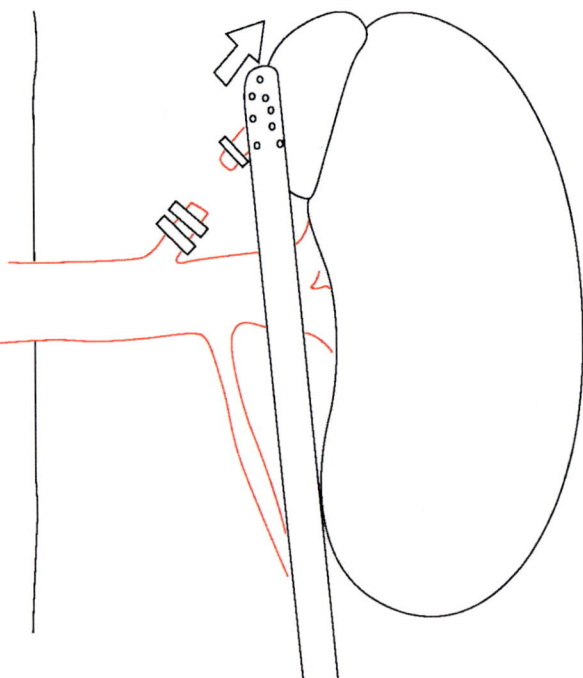

Fig. 10.1 Position of the left adrenal vein.

clipped and divided. At this point, the aim is to identify the psoas muscle immediately posterior to the clip and transected left adrenal vein. Thus, using an atraumatic grasper in the left hand, the adrenal gland is retracted anterolaterally and, using a hook electrode, the fibro fatty tissue along the inferomedial edge of the adrenal gland is divided until the psoas muscle is identified. Now all that remains is taking down the medial attachments of the adrenal gland to the aorta and the inferior attachments of the adrenal gland to the renal hilum. Occasionally, significant-sized adrenal vessels can be encountered which need specific attention. Thus, the key on the left side is to secure and transect the left adrenal vein, and identify the psoas muscle at that location thereby retracting the adrenal laterally and placing its remaining attachments on stretch.

On the right side, the key anatomic fact is that the right main adrenal vein exits the superomedial aspect of the adrenal gland and runs obliquely in a cephalad direction to enter the vena cava. Thus, the right adrenal vein is quite high immediately under the liver. As such, any smaller blood vessels encountered lower down along the medial aspect of the adrenal gland are likely not the main adrenal vein. The initial key aspect is to make the transverse peritoneotomy higher, 1 cm below and parallel to the undersurface of the liver (Figure 10.2). This will allow you to land on the adrenal gland directly. Thereafter, the right lateral edge of the inferior vena cava is visualized, the adrenal gland dissected and retracted laterally from it, and careful dissection performed in a cephalad manner to control the adrenal vein.

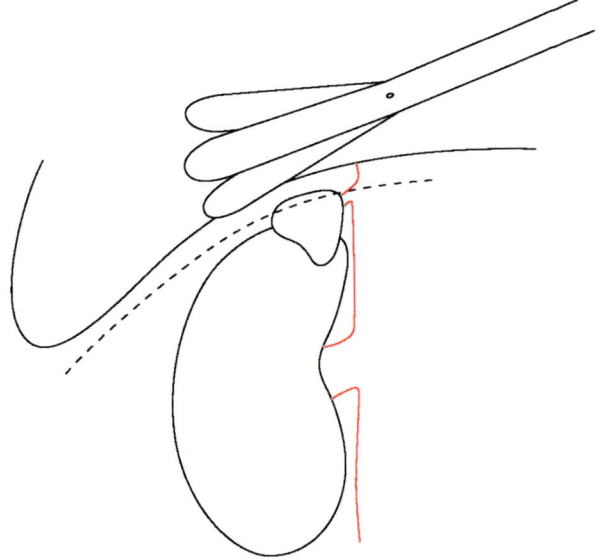

Fig. 10.2 Locating the right adrenal gland.

During Laparoscopic Adrenalectomy, How do You Identify the Adrenal Veins?

Dr. Ono

We have had only about 100 cases during the last ten years. We usually use the transperitoneal approach. On left side, we divide the peritoneum and then reflect the descending colon from the anterior aspect of the kidney and the renal vein is identified. This exposes the anterior surface of the adrenal and also leads us to the adrenal vein. We use medium-size metal clips across the adrenal vein before dividing it. On the right side disease also we use the anterior approach. We divide the peritoneum between the liver and the kidney and then make an additional incision alongside the inferior vena cava. The upper half of the kidney is exposed. The liver is retracted with a retractor. The renal vein is easily identified draining into the vena cava. Then dissecting along the vena cava to the liver, we can find right adrenal gland. It is important to identify the inferior vena cava first and also the right renal vein.

Any Tips for Laparoscopic Adrenalectomy?

Dr. Kaouk

The retroperitoneal approach is the approach of choice for adrenal masses with a significant retrocaval component.

Fat planes surrounding the adrenal mass should be inspected on preoperative CT or MRI. Presence of such surrounding fat is an indication of preserved planes and absence of local invasion to surrounding organs.

Dr. Stoller

During laparoscopic adrenalectomy, there is no need routinely to identify the adrenal artery. Adrenal arteries are usually arborizations of vessels that come from a variety of areas. In over 280 laparoscopic adrenalectomies, we have only identified a discrete adrenal artery two or three times that required formal ligation. The vast majority could just be dissected with a hook cautery or the harmonic scalpel.

When I do a laparoscopic adrenalectomy on the left side, I go from the upper left and come down and open it up like a book. On the right side, I dissect the upper edge from underneath the liver, going down to the vena cava and then clip the adrenal veins. On the right side, there is a 10% incidence of an aberrant adrenal vein coming directly from the liver into the adrenal. Therefore, on the right side one needs to be cautious, not of an adrenal artery, but of an aberrant adrenal vein going directly into the liver. It is important not to lose control of that vein but to use a harmonic scalpel or a formal clip ligation to secure it.

Additionally, for large adrenal masses that extend posterior to the renal hilum, one needs to be careful that one does not accidentally transect a segmental renal artery thinking that it is the adrenal artery. Adrenal arteries are the exception and not the rule and rarely need to be formally ligated.

Any Techniques and Tips for Partial Adrenalectomy?

Dr. Suzuki

When the tumor or lesion is located in the peripheral region of the adrenal gland, performing partial adrenalectomy is usually straightforward. Following exposure of the adrenal gland (there is no need to dissect or control the adrenal vein) we excise the mass lesion using the ultrasonic scalpel to divide the normal adrenal tissue. If bleeding is encountered, it can be controlled with bipolar forceps.

If a tumor is located close to the main adrenal vein, one can still perform partial adrenalectomy, as by preserving the superior adrenal veins/arteries, the function of the adrenal gland can still be preserved.

In patients with primary aldosteronism, recent reports suggest that in many cases, there is persistence of overactivity of the gland despite excision of the adenoma by partial adrenalectomy. This is felt to be due to the presence of microadenomas that may not have been appreciated on pre-operative imaging. We, therefore, have moved away from partial adrenalectomy in patients with primary hyperaldosteronism and instead perform total adrenalectomy.

Partial adrenalectomy is best indicated in patients with pheochromocytoma when associated with MEN type 2 disease (because of the high incidence of bilaterality in such cases).

Reference

1. Suzuki, K., Kageyama, S., Hirano, Y., et al.: Comparison of 3 surgical approaches to laparoscopic adrenalectomy: a nonrandomized, background matched analysis. J Urol **166**: 437, 2001

Chapter 11
Radical Prostatectomy

Which Do You Prefer: Transperitoneal or Extra Peritoneal Approach to Laparoscopic Radical Prostatectomy?

Dr. Li-Ming Su

I perform the classic Montsouris technique. I simply believe that this allows one to preserve the neurovascular bundle along its entire course with minimal traction in an antegrade direction. What I mean specifically is, during the Montsouris technique the seminal vesicles are dissected at the onset of the operation. By approaching the seminal vesicles in this fashion, one is able to virtually pluck the seminal vesicles out of their vascular bed and tease the nerve bundles off the seminal vesicles with excellent visualization, as there is minimal bleeding early in the operation. This is in contrast to the extraperitoneal approach, where the seminal vesicles are approached late in the dissection after the bladder neck has been divided. With this approach, one has to reach down and dig the seminal vesicles out from a hole with limited visualization, due to bleeding as well as urine in the field; and I am convinced that this is likely to result in more traction on the nerve bundles.

How Do You Identify the Bladder Neck During Laparoscopic Prostatectomy?

Dr. Eden

Try this. The most obvious guide is the shape of the prostate, and if you have a look at the lateral aspect of the prostate once the endopelvic fascia has been incised, you can follow the curve of the prostate medially (Figure 11.1). The next clue is where the fat adheres to the detrusor muscle, and that identifies the neck of the bladder. And if there is ever any doubt, one can always insert a

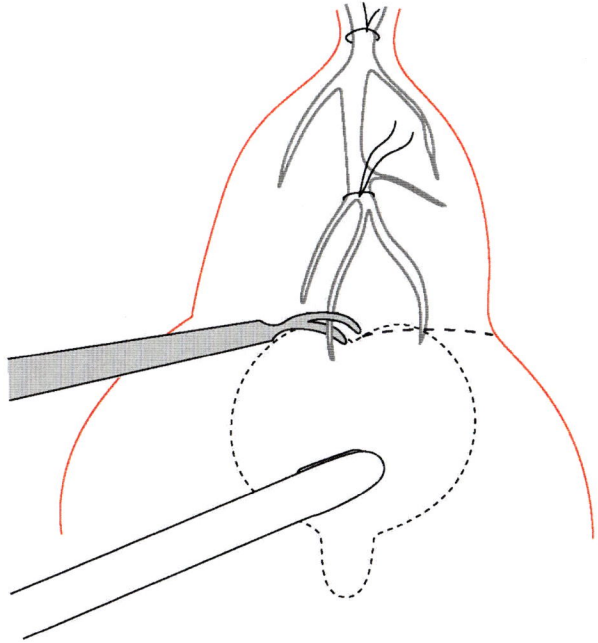

Fig. 11.1 Locating the bladder neck.

Foley catheter, if there isn't already one in there, inflate the balloon, and then pull back and that would clearly identify the bladder neck. It is always important to go more proximal rather than more distal. The last thing you want to do is to go into the prostate or risk leaving prostate tissue behind. Bladder neck reconstruction really doesn't take very long to do and even if you don't believe in bladder neck reconstruction, it is better to have a wider bladder neck and no prostate tissue left behind.

Dr. Gill

There is no 100% precisely definite way to identify the bladder neck during a laparoscopic prostatectomy. However, I tend to use three specific maneuvers:

1. The fat from the anterior surface of the prostate is peeled cephalad toward the bladder, thus exposing the prostate capsule. The point that the fat starts becoming more adherent and difficult to mobilize is typically at the prostato-vesical junction.

2. Back bleeding stitch is placed approximately 1 to 2 cm distal to the area where the fat becomes adherent. The tails of the stitch are left somewhat long. Anterior retraction is placed on the stitch, thereby retracting the prostate anteriorly. A transverse incision to divide the anterior bladder neck is made approximately 1 to 2 cm cephalad to this stitch.

3. A urethral dilator is inserted per urethra into the bladder. With the curved Bougie of the dilator facing

anteriorly, it is made to indent the bladder thereby showing the approximate location of the bladder neck. In my experience, use of the Foley catheter balloon to identify the bladder neck is not precise enough. Of course, we have been employing real-time transrectal ultrasound guidance to identify the bladder neck during a laparoscopic radical prostatectomy; however, this navigation tool might not be available at many institutions. A final point is that although in the past I used to make every effort to preserve the bladder neck, I no longer do so. Having a wider anterior cystotomy is not a major issue, and is preferable to making an inadvertent incision into the prostate thereby achieving a positive margin at the bladder neck. However, the posterior bladder neck incision has to be precise so as to preserve the ureteric orifices and get into the proper plane to mobilize the seminal vesicles.

How Do You Perform Nerve Preservation?

Dr. Eden

As far as nerve-sparing is concerned, I think the most important initial step, and this has got nothing to do with the so-called *veil of Aphrodite*, is to incise the lateral prostatic fascia high. Proximally, capsular vessels need to be clipped to allow this fascia to be divided without bleeding, but as the division extends distally, there is usually no bleeding. You need to incise this fascia all the way out to the apex and then gently push it down and what that will do is, display much more clearly the shape of the lateral aspect of the prostate and beneath it the lateral aspect of the neurovascular bundle. Once you've incised Denonvillier's fascia, you also have a very clear view of the medial aspect of the bundle. You then clip and divide the lateral pedicles of the prostate, staying close to the prostate and making no attempt at all to clip any vessels on the go side, in other words, from the prostate side. If there is a lot of back-bleeding, you can then put a clip on or use bipolar diathermy. The name of the game is to hug the prostatic fascia as far distally as possible. Because of the curve of the prostate, it is very difficult to complete the nerve dissection to the apex, and what I do is to leave the final one-third or so until after the dorsal vein complex and the urethra have been divided, and then it is much safer to take the apical branches coming off the neurovascular bundle and into the prostate. I think it is imperative that no energy source be used and certainly no form of monopolar cautery, no UltraCision, no Harmonic scalpel, and so on. What I do permit is the light use of bipolar cautery, if and only if there is bleeding from the neurovascular bundle that I absolutely cannot get a clip onto. I think it is also worth remembering that you can allow some bleeding from the neurovascular bundle as long as this is not arterial. Once you've got tissue apposition, in other words, once you've done the anastomosis, then you have the bladder pressing on the nerve bundles and you will then have exposed thrombin coming into contact with the blood, producing hemostasis. This part of the operation really has to be done very slowly.

Dr. Su

In terms of dissecting and preserving the neurovascular bundles during LRP, my preference is to perform a modified antegrade dissection of the neurovascular bundles. What is different about my technique is that before proceeding to the neurovascular bundle at the base of the prostate, I like first to release the nerve bundle along the lateral aspect of the prostate using a fine-tipped right angle dissector that has been modified to 0.8 mm in size. The key point is to identify the proper plane of dissection between the lateral pelvic fascia and the prostatic fascia. The neurovascular bundle lies between these two periprostatic tissue planes; so by incising the outer lateral pelvic fascia, this allows the surgeon to identify the neurovascular bundle and tease the nerve fibers away from the inner prostatic fascia. With this step, a lateral neurovascular bundle groove is developed. I believe that this lateral neurovascular bundle groove serves as an excellent landmark that guides the surgeon during antegrade dissection and preservation of the neurovascular bundles from the base to the apex of the prostate. Without dissecting the lateral neurovascular bundle groove early on, I think it is much more difficult for the surgeon to know precisely what direction or plane to take when dissecting the nerves in the antegrade direction.

With regard to the antegrade versus retrograde technique to neurovascular bundle preservation, I believe that the antegrade technique makes more sense, because it proceeds along the natural line of sight of the surgeon and it follows in line with the path of the nerve bundles from the seminal vesicle to the prostatic apex. The antegrade technique also allows for early ligation of the prostatic pedicle and late division of the dorsal venous complex, which are two major sources of bleeding. This results in minimal blood loss during the more difficult steps of neurovascular bundle preservation. As we need to have excellent visualization during nerve preservation, it is crucial to take the necessary steps to minimize ongoing blood loss that can obscure the proper plane of dissection and jeopardize neurovascular bundle preservation.

After releasing the nerve from the prostate as far distal to the apex as possible, the nerves are then released from the apex in a retrograde fashion after transecting the dorsal vein complex and urethra. By rocking the prostate apex in a cephalad direction, we can then tease the last remaining attachments of the neurovascular bundle, where it attaches to the apex. The apical dissection of the neurovascular bundle is typically the most challenging step as the nerve closely approximates the prostatic apex at the prostato-urethral junction. By leaving this step until the end after complete dissection of the prostate, the prostate is now more mobile, which helps to improve visualization of the precise course of the nerve bundles and facilitate their release and preservation at the apex.

How Do You Transect the Lateral Pedicle and Mobilize the Neurovascular Bundles During a Nerve-Sparing Prostatectomy?

Dr. Gill

We have developed a technique of transecting the lateral pedicle and sparing the neurovascular bundle that has

How Do You Identify the Bladder Neck During Laparoscopic Prostatectomy?

Dr. Eden

Try this. The most obvious guide is the shape of the prostate, and if you have a look at the lateral aspect of the prostate once the endopelvic fascia has been incised, you can follow the curve of the prostate medially (Figure 11.1). The next clue is where the fat adheres to the detrusor muscle, and that identifies the neck of the bladder. And if there is ever any doubt, one can always insert a

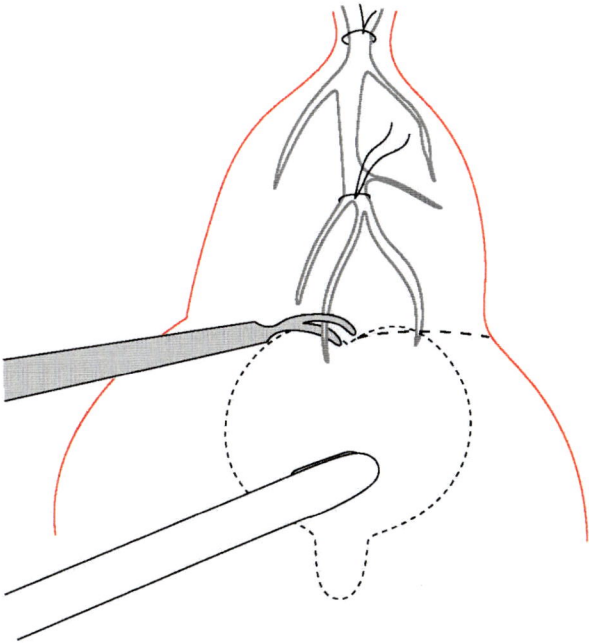

Fig. 11.1 Locating the bladder neck.

pedicle is obtained by precise, superficial hemostatic suturing with 4-0 Vicryl® suture on an RB-1 needle.

Any Tips for the Retrograde Nerve Sparing Technique?

Dr. Rassweiler

The first point I would like to make is that I prefer the ascending (or retrograde) technique as compared to the descending technique. The main problem of the descending technique is that when you cut through the bladder neck initially, you are not able to define the course of the neurovascular bundle (NVB). In contrast, in the classical ascending technique you identify the NVB from the beginning.

According to the fascial anatomy around the prostate, an interfascial dissection of the NVB should be carried out (i.e., between the levator and prostatic fascia). Recently, some authors (Menon et al., Gaston et al.) presented an intrafascial technique of dissection using an antegrade approach. In this method, the endopelvic fascia is not incised and the dissection of the prostate is carried out over the prostatic capsule. Evidently, this maneuver entails a high risk of positive margins and can only be used for early stages (i.e., T1c-tumors).

We divide the dorsal vein complex (DVC) to have optimal access to the urethra. Following adequate suture placement, we use bipolar coagulation in addition to dividing it step by step. Then at the apex we inflate a rectal balloon to identify the rectum and Denonvillier's fascia from the apex of the prostate. Additionally, it helps us to enlarge the dissection plane between the prostate and NVB without any traction on the bundles. It is crucial first to develop the triangle between the urethra and the apex of the prostate, thereby pushing the neurovascular bundle a little laterally and then coming down to the Denonvillier's fascia. You are then directly on the rectum.

After creating this space, you can create the groove between NVB and the prostatic fascia. If there are some small vessels, we clip them with 5-mm titanium clips. We do not use any bipolar diathermy or ultrasonic dissectors at this step. The only part where we use bipolar coagulation is on the prostate side.

When we have completely detached the apex of the prostate from the rectum and NVBs, we incise the urethra in a step-by-step maneuver: first the anterior wall is incised and the Foley catheter is retracted to identify the verumontanum. Then the posterior wall is transected distal to the veru under close endoscopic view to identify any prostatic tissue posterior to the urethra. Finally the posterior attachments between Denonvillier's fascia and rectum (i.e., recto-urethralis muscle) are divided. Usually the Foley catheter is sufficient to elevate the urethra. Alternatively, a special Rassweiler-bougie (Karl Storz) might be used.

After detachment of the urethra, the posterior dissection is carried out, following Denonvillier's fascia to the peritoneal fold (i.e., Douglas pouch), thereby detaching the rectum from the prostate. Only small branches from the NVB to the base of the prostate are clipped at this point.

Now we switch to an antegrade dissection starting at the bladder neck. We can very nicely identify the bladder neck by lifting the prostate up with the loop-like retractor of the divided Foley catheter. Having opened the bladder neck, we can identify the seminal vesicles and the vas after incising the Denonvillier's fascia posteriorly. The vas deferens is clipped and divided. The arteries feeding the seminal vesicles are also clipped at the tip of the seminal vesicle.

Anatomically, one has to identify three important structures at this point: the branches of the seminal vesicle artery, the proximal pedicle, and the neurovascular bundles. For this purpose you have to dissect the layer between the seminal vesicle and the proximal pedicle. This allows you to define the whole length of the proximal pedicle above the course of the neurovascular bundle.

According to the radicality of the procedure, you can go very close to the prostate or you can leave a small safety margin, which we usually do. All this is relatively easy, because one has already dissected the distal part of the neurovascular bundle down to the urethra and so, only the part closest to the seminal vesicles is yet to be dissected. Since the seminal vesicles have already been detached, again there is no problem. So the only thing that is still attached is the proximal pedicle which can be seen from both sides when elevated, and can be divided.

What Are the Optimal Angles of Port Placement to Facilitate Suturing in Radical Prostatectomy?

Dr. Rassweiler

It depends of course where one wants to suture and the technique one uses. I prefer to do my dissection from the

left side of the patient. I usually try to work with the ipsilateral two ports. The main point is that the ports should
not be too close together. I prefer not to use a semicircular line for port placement; instead I prefer a "W"
formation (Figure 11.3). If you place the ports, let's say,
near the umbilicus in a "U" or semicircular formation,
the distance between the trocars could be too narrow,
depending on the size of the patient and if too close then
they interfere with suturing. I got this suggestion from
Dr. Abbou.

Between the two ports that I use for suturing, the angle
is about 30 to 33 degrees, depending on the patient's size.
You need to have, for adequate suturing, an angle larger
than 24 degrees. I work with the left-sided ports as the
working ports for the dissection part and switch to the

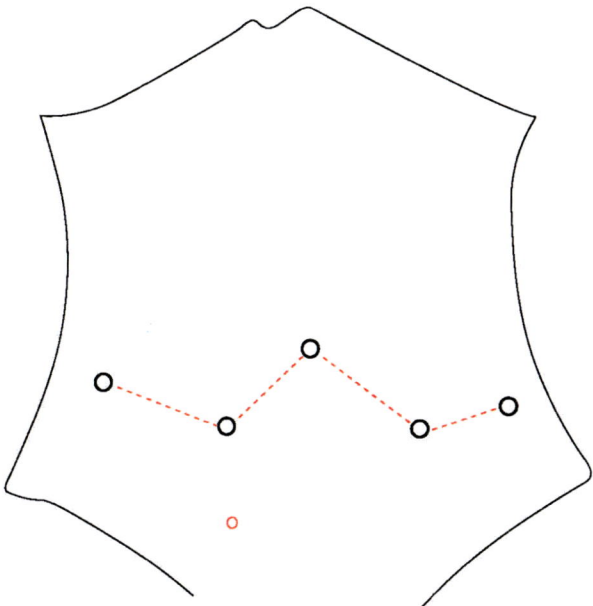

Fig. 11.3 "W-configuration" for port placement.

left lateral and the medial right port for the suturing part. The other trocars are then retracting the bladder neck or the bladder.

In our technique, we have an additional sixth trocar, because we use it for retraction of the balloon. I feel the addition of the sixth trocar improves the identification of structures, because I use it to lift up the prostate and in reconstructing the bladder neck (Figure 11.4). This nicely

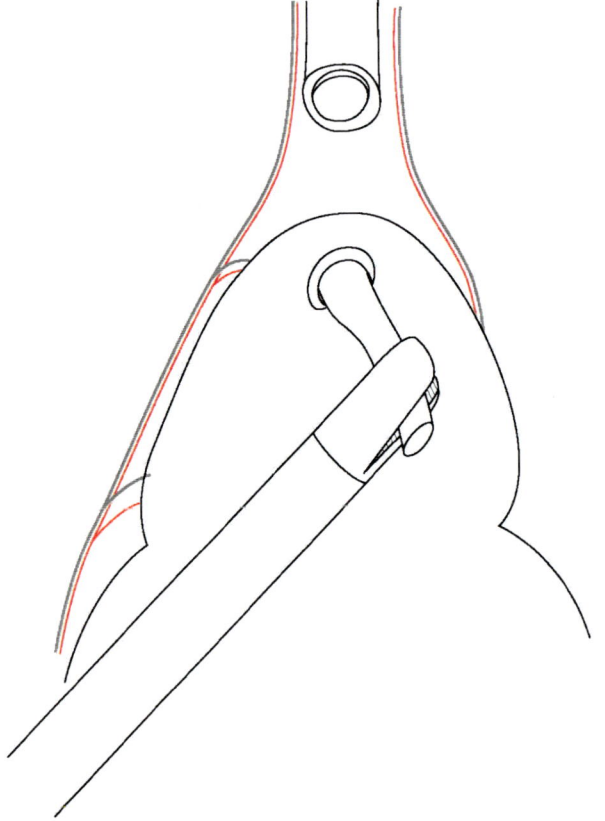

Fig. 11.4 Retraction of the apex of the prostate.

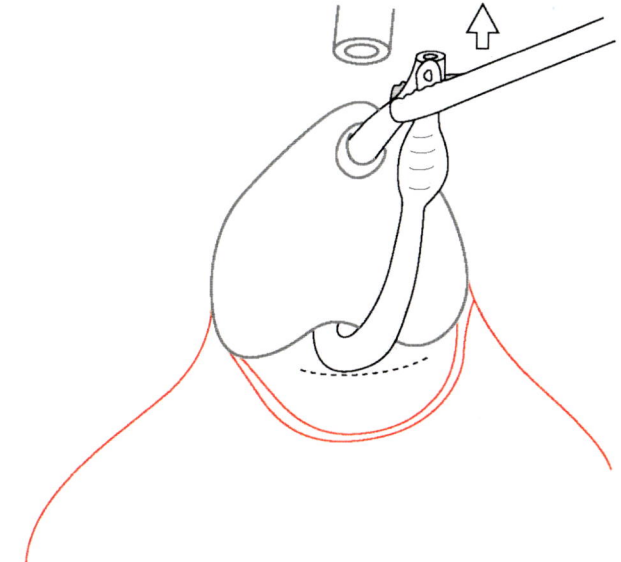

Fig. 11.5 Catheter loop retraction of the prostate.

displays the apex of the prostate or the bladder neck. It especially plays an important role in the latter part of our dissection, when we use the catheter as a loop-like retractor. The prostate is pulled up, and this trocar provides an excellent port for retraction (Figure 11.5).

How about Apical Dissection?

Dr. Kaouk

During apical dissection of the prostate, a laparoscopic right angle dissector is used to dissect a plane posterior to the urethra and just distal to the apex (Figure 11.6).

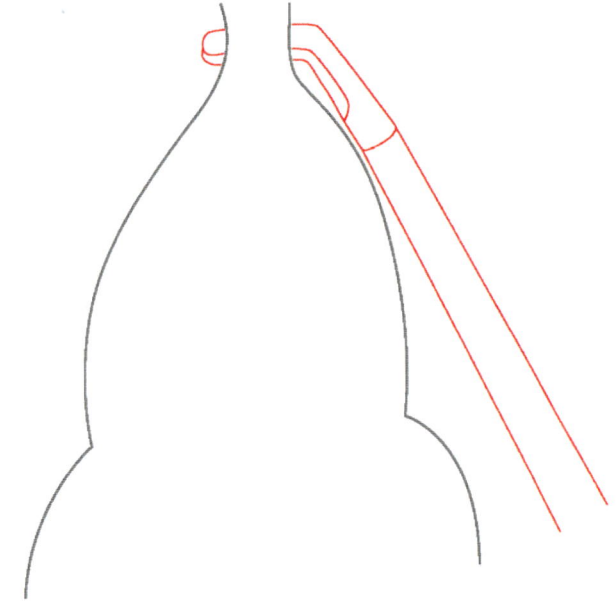

Fig. 11.6 Apical dissection with right-angled dissector.

This will minimize the chance of incising the posterior prostatic apex while transecting the urethra. However, generous dissection along the urethral stump toward the external urinary sphincter should be avoided, and the dissection should be limited to the point were the urethral incision is planned.

Dr. Rassweiler

Whenever you do nerve-sparing technique, you have to do a very adequate apical dissection. We do not perform nerve sparing when we have larger tumors or in cases of tumor in the apex. The tumor may have peri-neural invasion and may invade the neurovascular bundles. But you almost never have infiltration into the urethra. So I do the apical dissection first to find exactly the plane between the urethra and the dorsal vein complex.

Exposing the apex requires a rotational movement. Initially, the dorsal vein is fixed to the apex of the prostate. So after you suture ligate it (and usually I do a little bit of coagulation with bipolar, just enough to control the back bleeding), rotate the prostate. This is the main tip! In the beginning it appears attached but by cutting gradually down to the urethra, using a rotational movement, it is released. One has to be very careful in finding the layer between the prostrate, the urethra, and the dorsal vein complex. You have to be aware that the dorsal vein complex contains a middle part and usually two lateral parts that are also attached to the apical part. So you can suture the entire complex here but undermine the vessels, control them with bipolar diathermy, and then you have the prostate and the apex together. This is the anterior dissection.

The posterior dissection is performed when the urethra is exposed. You might be able to undermine the urethra, but you may injure the rectourethralis muscle. But when you do it with the right angle dissector, you always have to go toward the prostate. It helps to direct oneself with the balloon inside the rectum. Once you are on the rectum directly, it is a very safe layer. We then place a suture prior to complete transection of the urethra. I can then cut through the anterior wall of the urethra, lift the catheter, forming a little loop. The verumontanum is identified (which is my cutting line), and I then cut through with cold cutting. I cut through and once I get through the urethra I am at once in the right plane. This is the trick with apical dissection.

Of course, one worries about cutting into the rectum. With the above technique and with the balloon in the rectum, you know exactly where you are.

What Are Your Thoughts on Using an Energy Source During Dissection of the Neurovascular Bundles?

Dr. Su

There is now evidence from animal studies performed at our institution that any energy source—whether it be electrocautery or Harmonic scalpel—which emits heat energy should not be used in close proximity to the nerve bundles. The cavernous nerves to the penis consist of many delicate microscopic fibers that are closely applied to the prostate. Our canine studies evaluated the effect of energy sources used during dissection and preservation of the cavernous nerves on subsequent erectile responses. All of these energy sources, whether monopolar electrocautery, bipolar electrocautery or ultrasonic shears, resulted in significantly reduced erectile responses as compared to conventional nerve dissection without the use of energy. Survival studies performed at two weeks demonstrated no recovery of the cavernous nerves in the dogs. From this study, I believe that we can conclude that energy sources used in close proximity to the nerve bundles are likely to have a detrimental effect on cavernous nerve function and subsequent recovery following surgery.

With regard to nerve dissection, one other comment I would make is that in order to avoid electrocautery we use Hemoclips and cold transection of tissue, similar to what have been prescribed classically by Dr. Walsh in his open retropubic nerve-sparing approach, thereby avoiding the potential harmful effects of cautery or heat energy. The second issue is that in order to develop that precise plane that exists, which is virtually a potential plane between the nerve bundles and the prostatic fascia, one has to use better instruments. We are using macroscopic instruments currently to define a virtually microscopic plane. At our institution we have modified our dissectors, including the right-angle dissector and the curved dissector to a 0.8-mm tip design, thereby allowing us to perform fine dissection in teasing off the nerve bundle from the surface of the prostate. We have found that these tools are very useful in helping to preserve the nerve bundles and developing the precise plane.

How Do You Perform the Apical Dissection and Maximize Urethral Length?

Dr. Su

Similar to the bladder neck margin, I like to have a clear exposure of the apical margin. Therefore, I routinely divide the pubo prostatic ligaments by placing a urethral sound in the urethra and pressing down toward the six-o'clock direction. This maneuver tends to place the pubo-prostatic ligaments on slight tension, making them easier to identify and divide with either sharp dissection or with the hook electrocautery device. Dividing the pubo-prostatic ligaments allows the surgeon to place the dorsal venous complex stitch as distal and away from the prostatic apex as possible. This effectively increases the distance between the dorsal venous complex stitch and the apex, giving the surgeon plenty of room to divide the dorsal venous complex without compromising entry into the prostatic apex. In addition, it is very important to clean the apex of all the periprostatic fat before ligating the dorsal vein so that when you divide the dorsal vein you have a clear view of where the apex ends and urethra begins. Taking the same urethral sound and slowly drawing it backward, one can then identify precisely the plane where the urethra meets the apex, thereby maxi-mizing the amount of urethral length that can be safely left behind. It is critical to be cognizant of the fact that some patients have a posterior lip of prostate that may protrude underneath the urethra. Therefore it is impor-tant that the apex be cleaned as much as possible, so that a posterior lip of prostate is not left behind when tran-secting the urethra from the apex to the prostate.

How Do You Manage the Bladder Neck—Do You Preserve It or Not?

Dr. Su

There are studies that have indicated that with wider bladder neck resection you can reduce bladder neck pos-itive margins. These have been well demonstrated by Claude Abbou and his group. My preference is to take a slightly wider bladder neck margin and reconstruct it at the end with an anterior bladder neck closure. I do not feel that taking a wider bladder neck margin impacts on overall continence. Of note, our continence rate at one year is approximately 90%. I think that by making attempts to preserve the bladder neck one risks getting too close to the prostate, resulting in more bleeding and more importantly, the possibility of a positive bladder neck margin.

What Are Your Tips for Urethrovesical Anastamosis?

Dr. Kaouk

Significant bleeding from the neurovascular bundle after performing a nerve sparing radical prostatectomy may be controlled by applying Floseal® to the prostatic bed prior to performing the urethrovesical anastomosis.

Dr. Su

There are clearly many different techniques, all of which are probably equally efficacious. My preference, however, is the use of interrupted sutures. I like to start at the six-o'clock position outside-in on the bladder and inside-out on the urethra, establishing a nice posterior shelf by adding five- and seven-o'clock sutures (Figure 11.7). It is often helpful to have the assistant gently retract the bladder toward the urethra, thus reducing tension on these critical posterior sutures. Once this

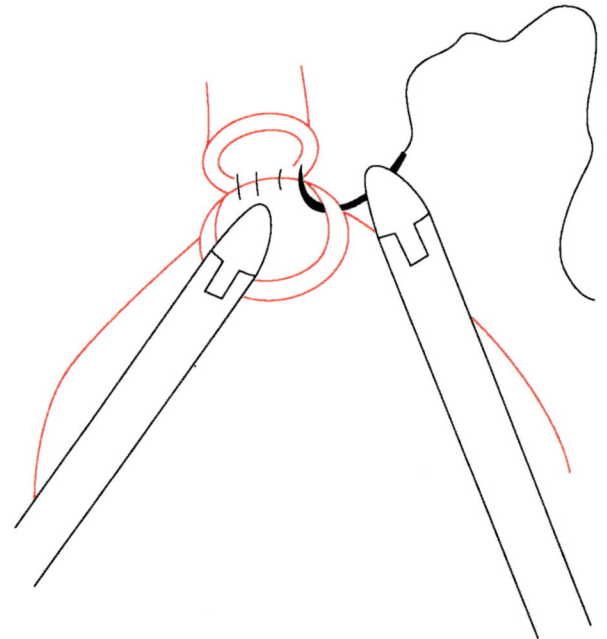

Fig. 11.7 Posterior anastomosis.

posterior anastomosis is completed, one can easily continue the interrupted sutures at the three- and nine-o'clock positions. When I reach the three- and nine-o'clock positions, I then take deep bites and close the anterior bladder neck, thus recreating a funnel-type effect of the bladder neck, which I believe improves continence rate, as it provides some resistance to outflow. Using interrupted sutures allows the surgeon to adjust for any discrepancies between the bladder neck and urethral opening. A running continuous suture has been described and used successfully by many. However, I think that this technique bunches up tissue and physically does not look as nice in my mind as compared to the interrupted sutures. In addition, a running suture requires that the assistant apply appropriate but not too aggressive traction on your suture while running the anastomosis. So one has to maintain constant attention to make sure that the assistant does not loosen the traction too much and allow the anastomosis to separate. On the other hand, overzealous traction results in tearing of the urethral side of the anastomosis.

Dr. Laguna

We like the single knot continuous suturing technique with two needles, going from the center of the posterior bladder neck (at the six-o'clock position) to the right with one needle and to the left with the other.[2] I think this saves time. We use Biosyn® (synthetic absorbable suture prepared from synthetic polyester Glycomer 631) 2-0 suture on SH needle. The length of suture you need is between 17 and 19 cm, depending on the width of the bladder neck. This allows about eight to ten stitches on either side. However, if you are planning to do an anterior tennis-racquet closure, you need an additional few centimeters, i.e., 20 centimeters of suture. The Biosyn® is available in two different colors (violet and undyed), allowing the use of different colors for the right or left side to avoid confusion.

Dr. Gettman

I use 2-0 Monocryl® suture on a urology needle as opposed to Vicryl because I believe this allows for the tissues to slide much easier. During the anastomosis, early on, I had some problems with urine leaks and found that if the bites were deep enough, almost burying the entire length of the needle into the bladder, that would provide me with adequate strength and completely eliminate the leaks. During the anastomosis, I like the assistant to provide perineal pressure, even if the urethral stump is no problem at all. It just seems like it helps set up the tissue better for the needle to be placed. Another thing is, when placing the needle in through the urethral side, I like to use a catheter that I have the assistant push in and pull out. I will insert the needle through the catheter and then pull that into the urethra and then dislodge it and that really sets up my needle throw through the urethra. I think that is a helpful step that I learned from Prof. Claude Abbou. The last thing is that, if there is a large bladder opening, or if the ureters are very close to the bladder neck, I like to do a Y-plication. This has been very helpful to drop the ureteral orifices at of harm's way. I do that with a 2-0 Monocryl® suture as well and then I use the standard tennis racket plication if the ureteral orifices are well out of harms way, but despite doing the running anastomosis, I found that having a smaller bladder neck facilitates achieving a water tight anastomosis. In fact, a smaller bladder neck allows the anastomosis to be performed in a running fashion with stitches anchoring the bladder at only the six-, three-, nine-, and twelve-o'clock positions.

How about Rectal Injuries?

Dr. Gettman

Thank goodness it hasn't happened to me more than once. I think it is important, even if you are over the learning curve, that you do bowel prep the evening before for all patients. What to do with the injury really depends on the extent of the injury and if there is actual fecal soiling. I think that it is absolutely reasonable to go ahead and repair this in two layers, using Vicryl® suture in the mucosa and then silk Lambert sutures. I think this can be safely performed laparoscopically or robotically, and if there's been bowel prep, then a diverting ileostomy is not indicated. However, I think that in all of these cases it is important to have a low threshold for seeking advice of a colorectal surgeon and also if there is any concern about the integrity of the closure, I think an open conversion should be recommended to make absolutely sure that there are no further sequelae from this injury.

References

1. Gill, I.S., Ukimura, O., Rubinstein, M., et al.: Lateral pedicle control during laparoscopic radical prostatectomy: Refined technique. Urology **65**: 23, 2005
2. Van Velthoven, R.F., Ahlering, T.E., Peltier, A., et al.: Technique for laparoscopic running urethrovesical anastomosis: The single knot method. Urology **61**: 699, 2003

Chapter 12
Robotic Prostatectomy

Any Tips for Trocar Placement for Robotic Laparoscopic Prostatectomy?

Dr. Gettman

Placement of a trocar two fingerbreadths above the pubic symphysis in the midline improves retraction during the procedure, especially with upward mobilization of the seminal vesicles and vas deferens. I also use stay sutures placed at the base of the prostate, so that the assistant can better retract the prostate via the suprapubic port. This allows for easier development of the recto-prostatic plane. The third trick that I like to use is to over-inflate the Foley catheter just prior to division of the prostato-vesical junction and then have the assistant intermittently pull on the catheter to help define the bladder neck. I found that by doing this I can initially start my dissection sharp and then with the other assistant providing superior traction on the bladder and the assistant using the catheter, pulling the catheter upward, that this plane will develop very easily.

Your Thoughts about Robotic Surgery?

Dr. Kaouk

All laparoscopic ports need to be spaced from each other significantly more than in regular laparoscopy to allow the bulky robotic arm the needed space for complete range of movement.

Although there is no tactile feedback, visual feedback for tension applied to tissue and suture line is an important compensatory factor.

The robotic needle holders' grip is significantly weaker than that of regular laparoscopic needle holders. The articulating tip should be utilized to optimize needle angle and minimize the torque force during suturing.

Check the rotational position of the needle holder prior to each needle pass to make sure that the needle holder has enough rotational range of motion. Otherwise, a 180-degree rotation of the needle holder in the opposite direction is needed to allow the full rotational movement of the needle holder during suturing.

In case of nonemergency conversion of a robotic case, laparoscopic surgery could be performed through the robotic ports depending on the reason for conversion.

In case of a dark-appearing field during robotic surgery, the most common reason is blood in the field that absorbs the light. So care must be taken to secure hemostasis and to suction the accumulated blood. In addition, the light source should be checked to increase intensity and the enhancement of the video setup should be increased.

What Are Your Thoughts about Robotics and the Future of Laparoscopic Prostatectomy?

Dr. Su

During the laparoscopic procedures performed at John Hopkins, we take advantage of the use of the AESOP robotic arm. My preference is to have a skilled, experienced laparoscopic assistant control camera movement using the hand-held remote control. Movement of the AESOP can be accomplished by using voice-activation, foot pedal activation, or remote hand-piece control. In my experience, movement of the camera is most efficiently performed by assistants who can follow commands of moving the camera left, right, up or down, and eventually, with experience, anticipate movements that the surgeon desires. Therefore I feel that this is the best way to perform laparoscopic prostatectomy in the most efficient manner and also it reduces the need for the assistant to hold the camera constantly, resulting in fatigue. With regards to the use of the da Vinci system, this is a fascinating robot that will only get better. My concern is that the current-generation device is a robot that was designed for cardiac surgery using cardiac surgery instruments. We must have a better selection of instruments specifically designed for prostatectomy in order to optimize, in particular, cavernous nerve preservation. Current techniques utilize a significant amount of electrocautery, which has been shown to affect cavernous nerve function adversely. But as we move forward in the field of endourology, robotics in the future will likely improve our abilities to accomplish more precise and perhaps more efficient surgery in a surgeon-friendly manner.

How Do You See Robotic Laparoscopic Prostatectomy (RLRP) to be Different from the Pure Laparoscopic Prostatectomy (LRP)?

Drs. Shalhav and Mikhail

With the evolution of the LRP technique, the addition of the robotic system has provided advantages and disadvantages as well as new challenges not previously encountered.

The robotic system offers many options not previously found in laparoscopic surgery. Some of these technological advances include 3-dimensional (3-D) view, increased instrument range of motion, tremor filter, and tele-surgical format. The 3-D view is achieved by the use of a double-lens scope embedded in a single 12-mm instrument attached to a heavy double-input camera. Although 3-D surgical goggles have been developed in an attempt to achieve 3-D vision during standard laparoscopy, these goggles are based on digital manipulation of an image received by a single camera, resulting in an artificial 3-D picture. With the improved visualization experienced in the robotic system, dissection of the neurovascular bundles and prostatic apex can be done more precisely than when standard 2-D laparoscopic vision is employed. In addition, the robotic camera is stable and rapidly guided by the console surgeon, unlike most pure LRP cases, where the camera is held by an assistant surgeon or a voice-activated system. In LRP cases where a robotic camera is not used, the assistant surgeon must constantly anticipate the surgeons' maneuvers and may be plagued with fatigue during prolonged cases, reducing the overall accuracy, which would be completely avoided with the robotic system.

Working in the pelvis during a radical prostatectomy, specifically with regard to creation of the urethrovesical anastomosis and knot-tying, provides a formidable challenge to novice laparoscopic surgeons as well as surgeons well versed in laparoscopic surgery. The learning curve is shortened and the ease with which these procedures are completed is significantly increased with the use of the robotic system. In addition to the 3-D view, the surgeon is afforded increased range of motion with improved degrees of freedom compared to use of the wrist. More recently, newer articulating laparoscopic needle drivers and other hand-held devices are being developed to mimic the range of motion achieved by the robotic arms.

The improved visualization along with the increased degrees of freedom the robotic system affords may be less advantageous for an experienced laparoscopic surgeon that has mastered the LRP. However, novice laparoscopic surgeons and surgeons without formal laparoscopic training may find these options invaluable. Ahlering et al. provides an example of an open surgeon that has now completed a large series of RLRPs with results equivalent to those of previously reported open and laparoscopic series.

The robotic system also has the capability of filtering out tremor, which may prove to be critical, especially when working with fine suture, such as during sural nerve grafting. At our institution we are currently performing robotic-assisted sural nerve grafting using 7-0 Prolene® with fine needle drivers when necessary.

Outside of open procedures, the surgeon is not able to palpate the capsule of the prostate directly. This limitation experienced during LRP and RLRP may be a hindrance in high-stage prostate cancer where nerve preservation would otherwise be optimized with direct tissue palpation. With regard to measuring suture tension, the surgeon can feel the transmitted forces during a LRP case, while the robotic surgeon cannot. However, over time the robotic surgeon can develop a visual perception for the amount of tension being placed on the suture as well as the force being applied by the instruments. This compensated perception of tactile forces is useful during a RLRP when handling or working near various organs such as the bowel or external iliac vessels during a lymph node dissection.

Lastly, the difference, between LRP and RLRP revolves around the availability of the primary surgeon. During an LRP, we can adjust the assistant's instruments as needed, especially when the assistant is less experienced with the case, while during an RLRP, the primary surgeon is very dependent on the laparoscopic skills of his assistant. The assistant has more responsibility to perform laparoscopic maneuvers without the direct manual guidance by the primary/senior surgeon. This arguably provides more laparoscopic autonomy for the assistant and encourages more independent skills training. However, if the assistant's laparoscopic skill set is still underdeveloped, the console surgeon is posed with an even greater challenge, especially in obese patients, where visualization and maneuverability are easily hampered by the patient's own body habitus as well as increased amount of intraperitoneal and pelvic fat.

What Are Your Techniques for Seminal Vesicle and Vas Deferens Release?

Drs. Shalhav and Mikhail

We typically start every robotic-assisted laparoscopic prostatectomy (RLRP) with a retrovesical dissection. Once the robot is docked, we begin retracting the sigmoid colon and rectum cephalad to expose the pouch of Douglas. Occasionally, the sigmoid is adherent to the left-lower abdominal wall, limiting its mobility. Therefore, more often than not, these adhesions need to be taken down to optimize exposure of the pouch of Douglas.

Identifying the location to open in the pouch of Douglas may require some trial and error until you become familiar with which ridge to open. Then you develop a gestalt on the location of the vas and seminal vesicles (SV). Also, the Foley can be manipulated to help identify the lower limits of the bladder. The peritoneum is then incised along the lower ridge seen in the pouch of Douglas, usually 1 to 2 cm above the rectum. We open the peritoneum widely to avoid working in a small hole. Judicious use of cautery and blunt dissection help locate the vas and SV bilaterally.

At this point, the first assistant grasps the anterior peritoneal flap with an atraumatic grasper, retracting the bladder anteriorly. Also the suction tip is used to retract the posterior flap toward the rectum. If anterior retraction of the bladder is difficult, check to ensure the bladder is decompressed completely. Without adequate emptying of the bladder, the bladder can inadvertently be injured or initially confused for the vas or SV during the early phase of one's learning curve.

Once the vas and SV are identified, we then proceed to dissect the SV off Denonvilliers' fascia with simple blunt dissection using minimal cautery. It is important during dissection of the SV to identify its primary arterial source near its tail and cauterize this using the bipolar grasper. Before complete dissection of the lateral surface of the SV, the vas is then mobilized about 3 to 4 cm and transected, avoiding too long of a tail, as this can later fall in front of the camera and interfere with your visualization. If the vas is not easily identified, the peritoneal opening can be extended toward the internal ring in order to identify the vas more distally. Once the vas is transected, the assistant then grabs the tail end and retracts it anteriorly toward the contralateral side. Therefore, it is important not to separate the vas from the SV completely, as this will limit the amount of SV retraction that you will be able to achieve at this point. Attention is redirected to the SV, which is then pulled medially using the bipolar graspers and blunt dissection with the spatula is used to sweep off the lateral attachments. Care is taken along the later aspect of the SV to avoid any thermal injury to the neurovascular bundles. Therefore, only limited bipolar energy is used until the SV is mobilized from its lateral attachments. Otherwise, the vas and SV are mobilized toward the base of the prostate.

After completing the dissection on one side, the assistant then retracts both the tail of the vas and SV anteriorly and laterally. Dissection is then carried out on the contralateral side in a similar fashion.

What Is Your Technique for Anastomosis During Robotic-Assisted Prostatectomy?

Dr. Shalhav

I use the Lapra-Ty® clip during completion of the urethrovesical anastomosis during a robotic-assisted laparoscopic prostatectomy (Figure 12.1). Although the robot has facilitated intracorporeal knot tying, I typically run my anastomosis from the six-o'clock to the twelve-o'clock direction. I use two separate 3-0 absorbable sutures cut to 6 inches and anchored together at their

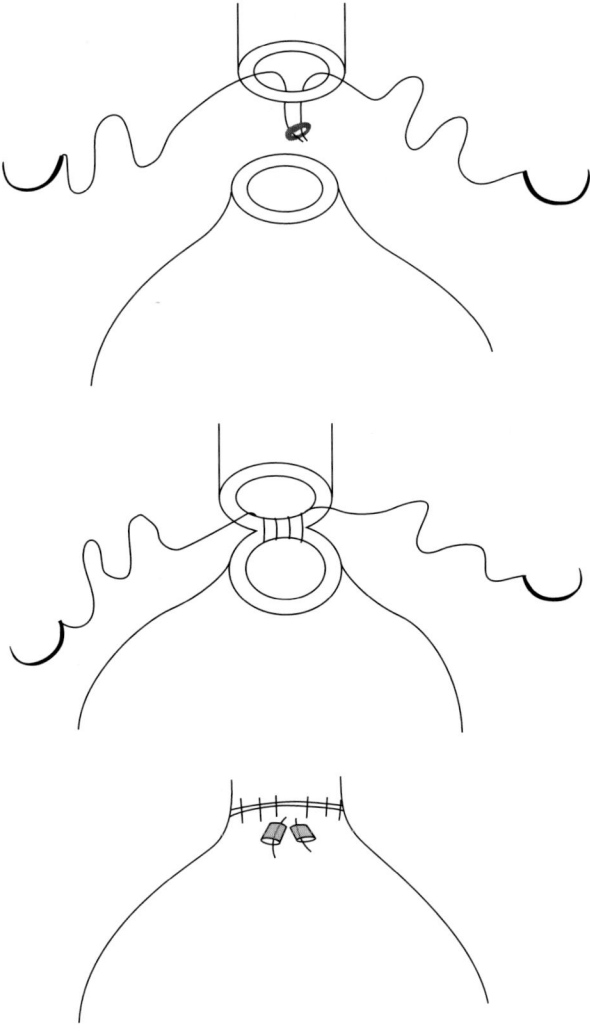

Fig. 12.1 Use of the Lapra-Ty clip for anastomosis.

tail ends using a Lapra Ty® clip. Each suture is run up to the twelve-o'clock position, where each suture is individually anchored using a Lapra Ty® clip. The benefit of this system is that if there is any slack in the suture line resulting in a leak, an additional Lapra Ty® clip can be placed in between the tissue and previous Lapra Ty® clip for further tension on the suture, thus resulting in better tissue apposition. However, it is important not to put too much tension on the suture line, as this can lead to ischemia and possible erosion of the Lapra Ty® clip through the anastomosis.

References

1. Ahlering, T.E., Skarecky, D., Lee, D., et al.: Successful transfer of open surgical skills to a laparoscopic environment using a robotic interface: initial experience with laparoscopic radical prostatectomy. J Urol **170:** 1738, 2003
2. Perer, E., Lee, D.I., Ahlering, T., et al.: Robotic revelation: laparoscopic radical prostatectomy by a nonlaparoscopic surgeon. J Am Coll Surg **197:** 693, 2003

Chapter 13
Laparoscopic Management of Ureteral Strictures

What Are the Technical Caveats for Laparoscopic Reconstruction for Distal Ureteral Strictures?

Dr. Desai

Iatrogenic injuries, both endoscopic and external, are currently the most common cause for ureteral strictures. Endoscopic treatment is the appropriate initial management option for short-segment strictures causing partial ureteral obstruction. Reconstructive procedures are reserved for strictures that are longer, obliterative, or that have failed endoscopic treatment. The reconstructive treatment options range from primary ureteroureterotomy, uretero-neocystostomy, psoas-hitch, Boari flap, and ileal ureter interposition, depending on the length and location of strictures. In select patients, these surgical techniques can be been performed laparoscopically with success.

We position the patient in a low lithotomy position, similar to other pelvic laparoscopic procedures. The port placement is similar to a laparoscopic radical prostatectomy. However, for distal ureteral re-implantation we typically use four ports (Figure 13.1). Additional ports can be added based on individual patient anatomy and stricture location to facilitate dissection, retraction, or suturing. We prefer percutaneous nephrostomy drainage over ureteral stenting preoperatively in patients that require some form of drainage. Ureteral stenting often causes significant inflammation and edema of the ureter and peri-ureteral tissues making reconstruction difficult. The initial step comprises identification of the normal, often dilated ureter proximal to the strictured segment. The iliac bifurcation is a reliable site for such initial ureteral identification. The healthy ureter is mobilized, maintaining the peri-ureteral adventitia until the ureter enters scar tissue. The ureter is transected at this point and no attempt is made to dissect the strictured ureter. Based on the length of stricture to be bridged, the ureter is implanted directly or via a bladder flap. We prefer to perform a refluxing ureteral re-implantation in all adult patients with stricture disease to minimize the risk of obstruction. For a direct uretero-neocystostomy, the ureter is implanted into an easily accessible area in the dome of the bladder. We prefer to place interrupted 4-0 Vicryl sutures on an RB-1 needle for the uretero-neocystostomy after adequately spatulating the ureter.

There are a few technical caveats for a laparoscopic Boari flap ureteral re-implant. Firstly, the bladder must

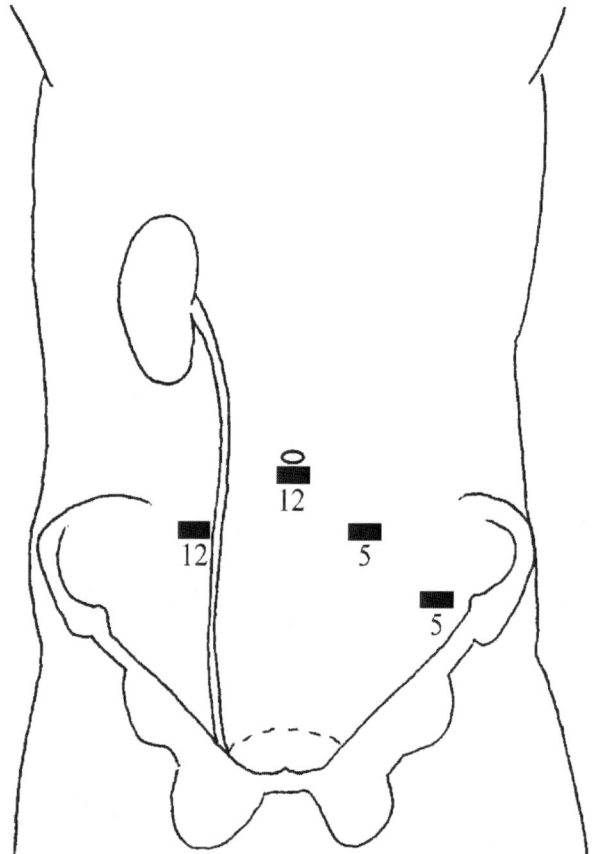

Fig. 13.1 Port placement for ureteral reconstruction.

be mobilized generously. Second, a large bladder flap must be fashioned, essentially incorporating the entire anterior wall (Figure 13.2). Lastly we make a mucosal trough on the apex of the bladder flap and suture the ventrally spatulated ureter to the trough on the bladder flap, creating a refluxing anastomosis.

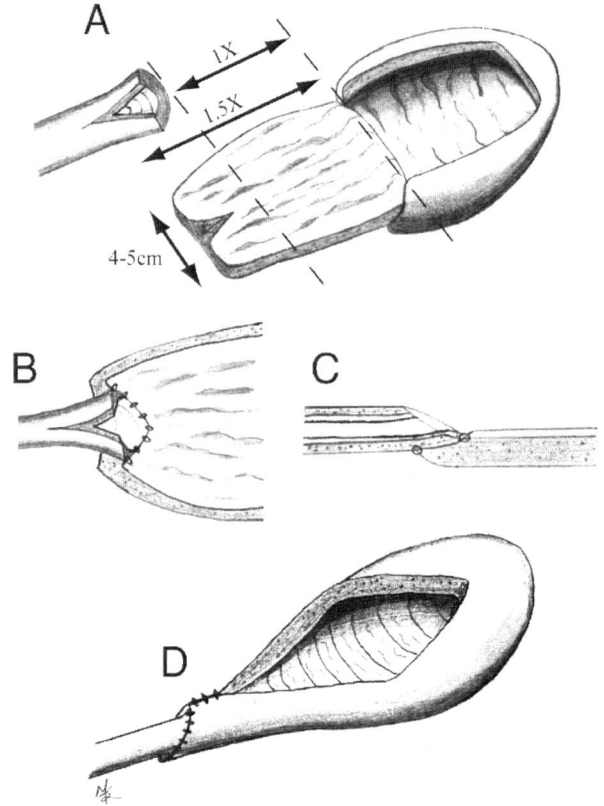

Fig. 13.2 Creation of Boari flap and anastomosis.

We place a 6 French JJ ureteral stent in all patients. For stent placement we insert a 2-mm trocar (Minisite, USSC, Norfolk, CT) in the suprapubic area. The 2-mm trocar is inserted such that the tip faces the spatulated ureteral lumen. Once the ureter has been anchored to the bladder with a few sutures, a Glidewire (0.035-inch straight wire, Microvasive, Natick, MA) is passed through the 2-mm trocar and then guided through the lumen of the ureter into the renal pelvis. The ureteral stent is threaded over the wire into the ureter. The Glidewire is then removed and the lower curl of the stent positioned into the bladder. The 2-mm trocar can be removed or left in place to facilitate suturing.

Chapter 14
Pediatric Laparoscopy

What Tips Can You Give Us about Pediatric Laparoscopy?

Dr. Alaa El-Ghoneimi

We are dealing with pediatric patients. Pediatric open surgical results are already excellent. So indications and results should be carefully assessed. There should be the least possible blood and nephron loss. In children, the space is very limited for trocar placement. Working space is also limited, especially when using the retroperitoneal approach. Monopolar diathermy should be used with extreme caution. We prefer using bipolar diathermy at all times.

As the space is very limited, especially in the retroperitoneal approach, the largest trocar we use is the 10-mm trocar. Even the 10-mm trocar should be avoided and substituted with a 5-mm trocar or smaller, whenever possible. This precludes the use of laparoscopic stapling devices. So one needs to master intracorporeal suturing and knotting techniques, as one may need to use such maneuvers even while performing laparoscopic nephrectomy.

While performing partial nephrectomy for duplicated systems, one needs to remember the differences in anatomy when compared to adults. There are duplicated vascular structures and ureters. During lower-pole nephrectomy, for instance, we place a ureteral catheter into the upper pole ureter, to enable us to inject methylene blue while dissecting the parenchyma (Figure 14.1). This helps recognize and treat any collecting system injury to the part of the kidney that is being preserved. The part of the kidney that is being preserved should not be dissected away from the peritoneum; this avoids the possibility of twisting of the renal pedicle, which can have disastrous consequences.

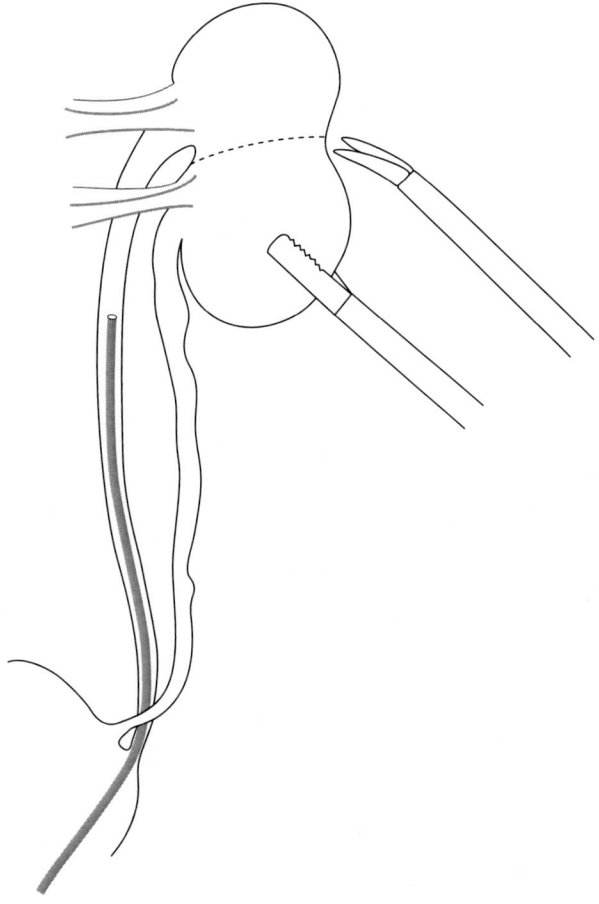

Fig. 14.1 Lower pole partial nephrectomy for duplicated system.

Are There Any Special Considerations during Laparoscopic Pyeloplasty in Children?

While embarking on reconstructive laparoscopic procedures in children, one should consider various points. First of all, the results of open pyeloplasty are excellent. The results of laparoscopic surgery should be equivalent to those of open surgery. Procedural modifications to dismembered pyeloplasty, such as Fengerplasty or V-Y plasty, which are designed to make laparoscopic reconstructions easier, have yet to prove their efficacy in the long term. In children, especially, who have longer life expectancies compared with adults, only time-tested techniques should be used. I would want the UPJ to be patent for at least 80 years!

In my own experience, I prefer to perform open retroperitoneal pyeloplasty in a child under 2 years of age as opposed to laparoscopic repair, as the technical difficulties are considerable and the morbidity of an open repair is minimal in that age group. A transperitoneal repair should be considered with caution in a child, as this creates scarring in the peritoneal cavity, which can have long-term consequences.

Port placement: The first port is placed at the tip of the 12th rib, and the two other ports are placed furthest away from this point, i.e., at the costa-vertebral angle and above the iliac crest.

We feel that the lateral approach to the kidney does not result in peritoneal tear, which I believe, happens during dissection of the kidney or ureter and not during the entry. To further reduce the risk of inadvertent peritoneal entry, one can place the initial access inside the Gerota's fascia behind the kidney, thereby displacing the kidney and with it the peritoneum anteriorly.

The suture material we use for laparoscopic pyeloplasty in children is an absorbable 6-0 suture. This suture can only be used in conjunction with a 3-mm needle driver. So in our setup we use a 3-mm trocar with 3-mm instruments. In retroperitoneal pyeloplasty the fourth trocar can be useful in retracting tissues or with holding tension on the sutures, but with experience we find the extra trocar more of a hindrance in the limited space available. In order to stabilize the suture line, we have found the placement of a stay suture at the UPJ anchored to the psoas muscle extremely helpful (Figure 14.2). The UPJ is kept stabilized with this suture until the suturing is completed, as it helps directing the scissors to make the spatulating incision in the ureter or the pelvis without physically handling the delicate tissues.

The standard drain we use is a double-J stent, but as its removal requires a second anesthesia, we often use a trans-anastomotic nephrostomy or pyelostomy. However, this is not possible, especially in cases with crossing vessels using the retroperitoneal approach, and in those cases we use the double-J stent. We place the stents in an antegrade fashion. This is particularly easy using the 3-mm trocars. The costa-vertebral trocar is ideally positioned to be in line with the anastomosis for easy insertion of the ureteral stent (Figure 14.3). Preoperative retrograde placement of the ureteral stent causes difficulties with the anastomosis, as it obscures the posterior suture line.

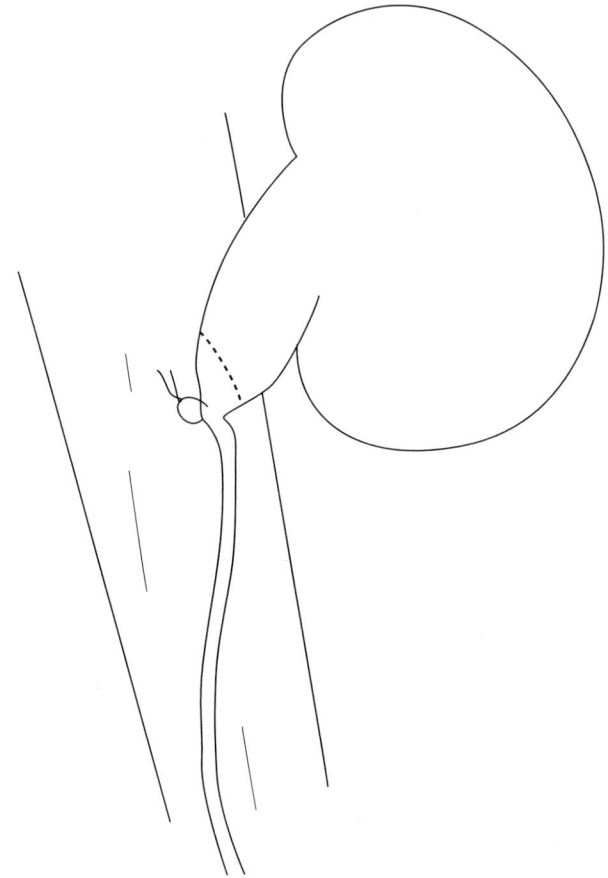

Fig. 14.2 UPJ anchored to the psoas muscle.

The length of the ureteral stent should be chosen carefully, as too long a stent causes discomfort to the child that negates many of the benefits of the laparoscopic surgery, and too short a stent may cause its retraction into the distal ureter! If one is doubtful, it is preferable to use fluoroscopy to guide the stent placement.

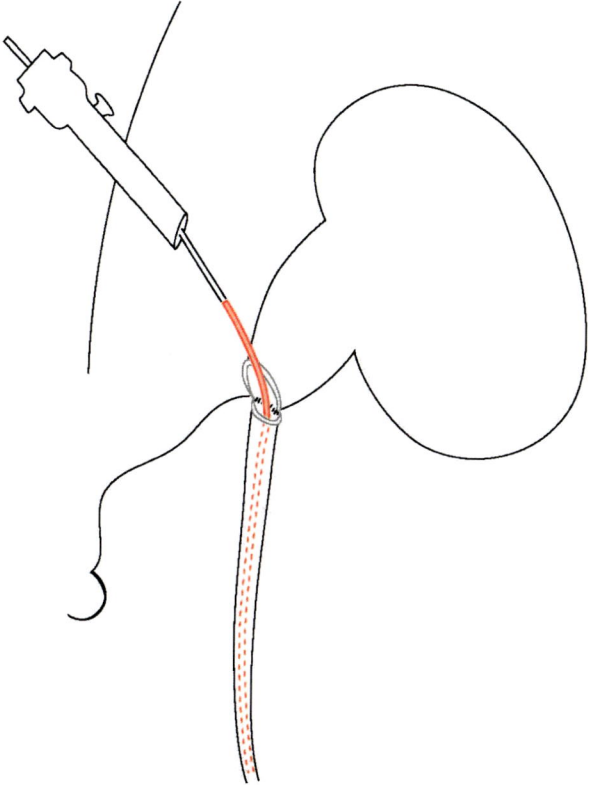

Fig. 14.3 Antegrade insertion of ureteral stent.

Any Contraindications to Pediatric Laparoscopic Surgery?

The experience of the entire operating team, including the surgeon, anesthesiologists, and nurses, should be taken into account when assessing the safety of performing laparoscopic surgery in children. While there are few contraindications for the experienced surgeon, surgeons performing transperitoneal surgery in children should be aware that complications such as those arising from bowel injury, etc., can be much more severe than those arising from the retroperitoneal approach. Intraperitoneal complications in children should be kept in mind at all times and suspected when there is high fever or abdominal tenderness. In such cases the abdomen should be explored at the earliest opportunity, as the results of a delay in diagnosis or treatment of even 6 to 12 hours can be disastrous in children. We should remember that more than ten years have elapsed since the beginning of laparoscopic experience in urology. The complications that were acceptable earlier on in the learning curve are no longer acceptable. Even experienced surgeons, when beginning a novel procedure, should not hesitate to consult with other surgeons or colleagues more knowledgeable with the particular procedure. They will never regret this.

A word of caution: in retroperitoneal surgery orientation is paramount. Frequently check your landmarks, i.e., psoas, kidney, and peritoneum. If one is not careful, the inferior vena cava can be mistaken for the renal vein because of improper orientation. If one encounters bleeding from the renal pedicle, place the pedicle on tension by elevating the kidney. Then carefully assess whether it can be controlled laparoscopically or if it needs conversion to open surgery. Do not rush while converting to open surgery. Maintain the pedicle on tension to minimize bleeding when converting to open, as significant bleeding even for a few minutes in a child can be fatal.

I have a criticism of the current practice of "video-assisted pyeloplasty," wherein the pelvis and ureter are dissected laparoscopically, delivered outside, the repair is performed in an open fashion, and then the anastamosis delivered back into the retroperitoneum. One should either perform open pyeloplasty, which has near-perfect results, or be able to perform the entire surgery in a laparoscopic fashion to achieve equivalent results.

One more point for consideration! Just as no one would consider himself competent to perform hypospadias surgery merely because he has done over a thousand circumcisions (as it requires years of training to understand the anatomy and the nuances of reconstructive pediatric surgery), one should not undertake major laparoscopic ablative or reconstructive surgery unless one has invested equivalent training in acquiring the requisite skills.

Chapter 15
Complications

What Are You Thoughts about Laparoscopic Complications?

Dr. Cadeddu

In preparation, whether one is doing a simple nephrectomy or a more complex case, I think one always has to be prepared for complications, the most significant being vascular and bowel-related. As far as vascular injuries are concerned, I always have my laparoscopic suture instruments and the laparoscopic applicators available in the room, not necessarily open, but they should always be in the room. The nice thing about the Lapra-Ty® is that you can get a 5–6-inch length of suture and put a Lapra-Ty on the end of it and you can rapidly sew and follow yourself. For example, let's say you lacerate the gonadal vein. One important thing, I think, is always to be aware of the colon during kidney and adrenal surgery. Colonic injuries can be devastating. The presentation of a patient with a bowel injury is distinctly different from the presentation of a patient after open surgery. A patient with bowel injuries due to laparoscopic surgery tends to present with unique symptoms. They generally do not have peritonitis, but what they do tend to complain about is pain localized to one trocar site. No one, I think, understands this particular point. They tend to have leukopenia, not leukocytosis. They usually have leukopenia with a left shift. They can have diarrhea instead of an ileus, but they often have nausea and vomiting and they may be afebrile. So if a patient has an atypical recovery and these signs and symptoms have been found, it is very important to identify a bowel injury. Drs. Jay Bishoff and Louis Kavoussi published an article describing these series of presentations. Having had my own experience with bowel injury, I can tell you it is absolutely true.[1] Evaluation of bowel injuries when suspected postoperatively should start with a CT scan. Even if the CT scan is negative on day 1, if you still feel concerned, sequential serial CT scans looking for an abscess or free air are required.

How Do You Deal With a Splenic Injury?

Dr. Wolf

For a splenic injury, the argon-beam coagulator is the best coagulating tool and will work well for most minor injuries. For a larger injury, one that does not stop bleeding with the argon-beam coagulator, we use a fibrin glue/gelatin sponge composite (Tisseel® and Gelfoam®) for hemostasis (see partial nephrectomy section). This is most effectively applied with hand assistance, so if we don't have a hand in, then we will usually use a slurry of thrombin and gelatin granules (Floseal®). Conversion to hand assistance to control splenic injury is not unreasonable, and that might be better than taking the spleen out. In same cases, of course, the splenic bleeding cannot be controlled and splenectomy will be required. If you do a lot of laparoscopic procedures on the left kidney, especially radical nephrectomies for large tumors, you will need to address splenic injuries and on occasion will have to do a splenectomy. The urologist should be able to do the splenectomy in this situation, which is straightforward for a normal spleen, especially with hand assistance.

Dr. Gill

As with any other complication, the best strategy is not to cause such an injury in the first place, by adhering to some of the points mentioned earlier (see general laparoscopy). If an injury does occur, a careful evaluation has to be made to determine the extent of the injury and its potential for immediate as well as delayed complications such as hemorrhage and bile leak. If there is any question, a general surgery intraoperative consult should be obtained. More typically, for the liver, using an argon-beam coagulator at a setting of 120 to 150 watts will achieve adequate hemostasis rather easily. A deeper laceration may require suturing of the liver parenchyma. This should be performed after consultation with the general surgeon. A splenic injury is a more serious problem. If not addressed adequately it can have serious sequelae. A superficial injury such as a capsular tear or a superficial splenic laceration may be adequately controlled with precise argon-beam coagulation with topical application of Floseal and pressure with Surgicel.® Observation of this area for 10 to 15 minutes at a lower pneumoperitoneum is important to confirm hemostasis. A deeper splenic laceration is not likely to be controlled by the above measures, and they require a splenectomy. General surgery consult must be obtained.

How to Handle Diaphragmatic Injuries during Laparoscopy?

Dr. Suzuki

One should be vigilant during surgery of the adrenal and upper pole of the kidney. If there is a tear in the diaphragm, the carbon dioxide gas enters the pleural cavity and causes paradoxical movements of the diaphragm. If one observes unusual movement of the diaphragm during surgery, carefully look for tears in the muscle; if present, they can be repaired by suturing.

How Does One Manage an Intraoperative Pneumothorax?

Dr. Gill

An intraoperatively detected pneumothorax typically occurs following an inadvertently created rent in the diaphragm. As such, the diaphragmatic opening is immediately visible, and may be associated with increasing difficulty in ventilation per the anesthesiologist. Typically, such a diaphragmatic injury occurs during renal or adrenal surgery. If the patient is stable from the ventilation standpoint, we do not repair the diaphragm immediately, preferring to defer repair until the end of the primary laparoscopic procedure. Typically, this is the case. Depending on the size of the diaphragmatic rent, we typically carefully employ a CT-1 needle with 2-0 Vicryl® to place a precise figure-eight stitch to re-approximate the diaphragmatic rent. Care must be taken not to incorporate lung tissue in the stitch; otherwise a broncho-pleural air leak will result. Prior to tightening the figure-eight stitch, a 12 or 14 French red rubber catheter is inserted through a 5-mm port site through the abdomen into the diaphragm rent and the pleural space. The external end of the catheter remains outside the body and is placed under water to create a water seal. The ends of the figure-eight stitch are tightened. The pneumoperitoneum pressure is reduced to 5 mm Hg, and the anesthesiologist is requested to give 10 to 15 large insufflations through the ventilator so as to completely expand the lung, thereby driving out the pleural air through the catheter into the water seal. Concomitantly, the figure-eight stitch is tied down and the catheter is pulled, thereby achieving an airtight repair. On occasion, the diaphragmatic rent may be larger and not amenable to primary re-approximation. In such instances, we have employed a tailored Dacron graft, which is sewn in to the diaphragmatic opening. Incidental pneumothorax detected postoperatively on chest x-ray typically requires no management if the pneumothorax is less than 30% of the ipsilateral pleural space, and the patient is hemody-namically stable and oxygenating well. Given that the pneumothorax is composed of Carbon Dioxide, sponta-neous reabsorption is the rule. However, if cardio-respiratory compromise occurs, a chest tube can be placed in the recovery room.

How Do You Handle Vena Caval Injury?

Dr. Kavoussi

The first thing to do is apply pressure; for small tears in the vena cava, pressure plus local Floseal® application, should be sufficient. One should hold pressure for 5 to 10 minutes with a gauze pad. In case of a small venotomy, just pinching the vena cava in that area and placing a row of titanium clips can secure hemostasis. Alternatively, the venous injury can be over-sewn with laparoscopic free-hand suturing. One can place a Weck® clip or Lapra-Ty® clip on the end of the suture instead of a knot and then use that to run a figure-8 stitch to close the vena cava. Alternatively, an Endostitch® device can be used. One should be careful to maintain adequate lumen of the vena cava, but 80–90% of the smaller injuries of the vena cava can be controlled with pressure alone. Of course, having adequate laparoscopic experience and expertise is essential, and open conversion should always be kept in mind. Also, before exiting, the site should be inspected after 5 to ten minutes of desufflation.

Are There Any Tips Regarding Avoiding Injury to the Superior Mesenteric Artery during Laparoscopic Renal Surgery?

Dr. Gill

The superior mesenteric artery (SMA) has occasionally been injured during laparoscopic left radical nephrectomy or left adrenalectomy for a large adrenal mass. Remember that the SMA is intimately related to the cephalad edge of the left renal vein, anterior to the aorta. Thus the left renal vein is located in the angle created by the SMA with the aorta. During transperitoneal laparoscopic renal/adrenal surgery, we take care to stay lateral to the left lateral border of the aorta and anterior to the psoas muscle during dissection of the renal hilum. Care should be exercised when controlling the left renal artery and vein, especially in the presence of prior scarring or adhesions. When excising a large left adrenal mass, meticulous care must be taken along the medial aspect of the tumor to avoid dissection straying medially anterior to the aorta. Finally, during a transperitoneal left live donor nephrectomy, the left renal vein is often mobilized and stapled at the inter-aorta-caval region, in order to maximize renal vein length. During this maneuver, it is important not to advance the Endo-GIA stapler too far cephalad, in an attempt to encompass the renal vein completely within the stapler jaws. Doing so may inadvertently advance the stapler too close to the origin of SMA. Therefore, we typically transect the left renal vein only across its partial circumference/diameter and complete the venous transection by clipping and dividing the remaining vein segment.

Retroperitoneoscopically, the left renal artery is the first vascular structure visualized during left radical nephrectomy. As such, it is usually quite clear and no confusion exists about its identity. However, on occasion, especially in the setting of multiple left renal arteries, one can have confusion about the identity of a cephalad-arising renal artery. Again, the best strategy is to mobilize this vessel circumferentially without clipping it. The remainder of the kidney is now completely mobilized and retracted laterally. As in the transperitoneal approach, if the previously mobilized blood vessel is heading directly into the kidney, it is confirmed to be the renal artery and is clipped and transected. On the other hand, if it is not heading toward the kidney, it is the superior mesenteric artery and is left as it is. Superior mesenteric artery injury is a major vascular complication obviously, which can be fatal.

How Do You Handle Carbon Dioxide Gas Embolism?

Dr. Gill

CO_2 embolism is a rare event, and I have personally never seen it in more than 3,000 laparoscopic cases. However, it can occur as a result of direct infusion of carbon dioxide into the vascular system or excessively high pneumoperitoneum pressures for a prolonged period of time. Typically, a precipitous increase in end-tidal Carbon Dioxide and decrease in end-tidal O_2, accompanied by hypotension are the initial warning signs. Immediate desufflation of pneumoperitoneum is mandatory. Occasionally, a mill-wheel murmur is detected by the anesthesiologist. Ventilator adjustments are made by the anesthesiologist to stabilize the patient. Occasionally, aspiration of carbon dioxide bubbles from the heart is necessary through a central catheter placed within the superior vena cava.

How Do You Handle Some Unexpected Internal Abdominal Bleeding, for instance, during a Nephrectomy?

Drs. Shalhav and Mikhail

The best method is prevention. We are firm believers in immediate control of even the slightest of bleeding. A bloody surgical field is a dark one with poor vision that promotes errors. In order to prevent a major bleed you must keep a pristine surgical field, with careful dissection and optimal exposure. It is important to optimize your exposure even if that means adding an additional port for retraction. To prevent unwanted bleeding from the inferior epigastric artery, avoid trocar placement through the rectus muscle. Therefore, medial ports are placed either through the linea alba in the midline or along the para-rectus line, about 7 to 10 cm lateral from the midline.

Our typical port placement includes using four ports on the left side and five on the right. On the left side, the left arm and camera ports are along the left para-rectus line with the right hand and second assistant ports located one or two fingerbreadths above the level of the umbilicus along the anterior and mid-axillary lines, respectively. In our opinion, this port configuration allows for optimal view of the renal hilum which is essential when dissecting the renal artery and vein. Occasionally, in obese patients an umbilical port may be used for retracting bowel for optimal hilar exposure. With regard to a right-sided procedure, the left-sided port placement described above is mirrored on the right side with everything lowered one or two fingerbreadths. Otherwise an additional port is placed in the midline at the level of the right-hand port to serve as a liver retractor. These port configurations triangulate toward the renal hilum on either side, again optimizing visualization and dissection of the hilar vessels.

Another useful preventive measure is to evaluate the hilar vasculature as well as possible using preoperative imaging. It is helpful to know if there is more than one renal artery or vein. In addition, on occasion, one could identify large lumbar veins emanating from the left renal vein. In our experience, we have also encountered anomalies such as retro-aortic renal vein, a branch of the right renal artery traveling anterior to the inferior vena cava, as well as a left inferior vena cava which were not noted on the radiology report and were helpful to know about during the hilar and peri-hilar dissections.

During surgery, we have different ways of controlling bleeding depending on its severity. When bleeding occurs, we immediately increase the pneumoperitoneal pressure to 20 mm Hg to create a tamponade phenomenon. We ensure that our gas flow is maximally set to 40 liter/minute to ensure that we maintain adequate intraperitoneal pressure, especially in the presence of aggressive suctioning. In addition, we use direct pressure either by the suction tip or a Kittner which is held by the assistant. Pressure is held until adequate suctioning and visualization are achieved. If the bleeding is minimal, after the above measures have been taken, many times you can leave this area to work in another area and the bleeding will have stopped in the interim.

If bleeding continues and is not from a vessel, there are numerous thermal and nonthermal measures that can be used to obtain hemostasis. If bleeding is encountered from parenchymal organs such as the liver, spleen, or adrenal gland, this could usually be controlled by thermal methods using bipolar cautery, ultrasonic shears, or argon beam coagulation. Small vessel bleeding can also be controlled by these methods. Also, these bleeding sites can be controlled with intracorporeal suturing and bolsters. Specifically, we have encountered two renal vein injuries that we were able to repair intracorporeally using 5-0 Prolene® suture in a figure of 8 fashion both times. Otherwise, for larger vessels such as the external iliac vein, we have repaired the laceration quickly using 3-0 Prolene suture with a Lapra-Ty® on each end eliminating the time needed tie each knot intracorporeally. One thing to note is that we are always ready to convert to an open procedure, especially if the bleeding is too brisk or very difficult to manage intracorporeally. Judgement is key; you need to give yourself a little time to realize if this repair is going to work laparoscopically. Our rule of thumb is that if the patient will require a blood transfusion by the time we would be able to repair the vessel injury, then we should convert to an open procedure.

When significant bleeding is encountered from a renal hilar injury, an effort should be made to repair it. However, when repair is not possible or the bleeding is too brisk and the vein and artery are satisfactorily dissected, then we use an Endo-GIA stapler (Autosuture, Norwalk, CT) temporarily to occlude the renal hilum en bloc. If bleeding is controlled, an attempt at repair should be made. If repair is unsuccessful or not feasible and care has been taken not to staple inadvertently across the aorta, inferior vena cava, adrenal gland or the pancreas, the hilum is then divided en bloc. Very rarely, the renal vein can be transected prior to the renal artery. With the renal vein ligated first, the kidney becomes engorged and oozy and dissection of the renal artery becomes even more difficult. Otherwise, there is the theoretical risk of opening collateral channels with an increased risk of metastatic spread. It is also important when using the stapler to ensure that no surrounding clips have been incorporated into the staple line as this could lead to dysfunction of the stapling device.

Again it is worth mentioning the importance of maintaining a low threshold for open conversion in the presence of bleeding. It is important to gain control early without having lost massive amounts of blood. In the end there is no shame in an open conversion, but rather satisfaction in knowing that you used proper judgment.

Lastly, there are hemostatic agents that are available on the market such as thrombin matrix, fibrin glue, and cellulose. All of these products can be used in a laparoscopic field; however, we do not rely on these agents to obtain hemostasis and therefore use these items on a limited basis. FloSeal® is only applied over the resection bed during partial nephrectomy and into the tract of the cryo probe after its removal following a cryoablation. Otherwise, we do not typically use hemostatic agents on a routine basis.

How Do You Handle an Inferior Epigastric Artery Bleed during Trocar Placement?

Dr. Shalhav

Again the best way to handle such injuries is to prevent them. As was mentioned above, I typically place my medial ports in the midline or along the lateral aspect of the rectus muscle which is about 7 to 10 cm lateral to the midline. In the past, I have had a couple of these injuries; however, at the current rate of over 200 cases per year, I have not had this problem with the above port configuration.

Now, intraoperatively, epigastric vessel injury is easily recognized when significant oozing is seen usually in a pulsatile fashion around the trocar. When epigastric arterial injury is identified, it can easily be controlled via an intracorporeal approach. One thing to keep in mind, is the cranial to caudal direction of the epigastric artery, and therefore it needs to be controlled above and below the trocar site.

First of all, the trocar should be left in place. I typically deal with these bleeds right away rather than wait until the end of the case. I use an intracorporeal technique where I use a 2-0 Vicryl suture on a CT1 needle cut to 4 inches with a Lapra-Ty® clip on its tail end. I throw a figure 8 stitch above and below the trocar site with the port still in place. I anchor each proximal end of the suture with a Lapra Ty® clip as well. I then temporarily remove the port to ensure hemostasis has been achieved. Once this has been done, I replace the port through the same site and proceed with the case as scheduled.

One of the biggest tips I can give is related to the use of the Lapra Ty® clip. As stated earlier, Lapra Ty® clips obviate the need for knot-tying which can be imperative when time is of the essence particularly when repairing a vascular injury. With a Lapra Ty® clip, a clip is placed on the tail end; and once the suture has been run, a second clip is placed on the proximal end after appropriately cinching down on the tissue. If for any reason, the suture is too loose, a second Lapra Ty® clip can be placed underneath either end to further tighten the suture line.

Reference

1. Bishoff, J.T., Allaf, M.E., Kirkels, W., et al: Laparoscopic bowel injury: Incidence and clinical presentation. J Urol **161**: 887, 1999

Index